Piet G de Boer

Orthopedic and Trauma Surgeons: CPD in Community Hospitals

A study of different educational needs and preferences

The author

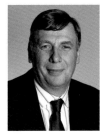

Piet G de Boer, MA, FRCS

Piet de Boer was educated at Downing College Cambridge in the field of experimental psychology and received orthopedic training from St Thomas' Hospital London. In the early 1980's, while in New York as visiting Professor at Yeshiva University, he co-authored the best seller Surgical Exposures in Orthopaedics with Stanley Hoppenfeld, which is now in its 4th edition. Awarded an AO Fellowship in Tubingen, Germany in 1984, Piet de Boer went on to work as a consultant orthopedic surgeon in York for 20 years.

Appointed the first Director of Education for the AO Foundation in Davos Switzerland in 2006, he is currently an Honorary Senior Lecturer at the Hull and York Medical School in the UK, and a visiting lecturer to the University of Rijeka in Croatia.

He has published many articles in peer reviewed journals, authored four other successful books in the fields of orthopedics and education, and is currently working on his first detective novel.

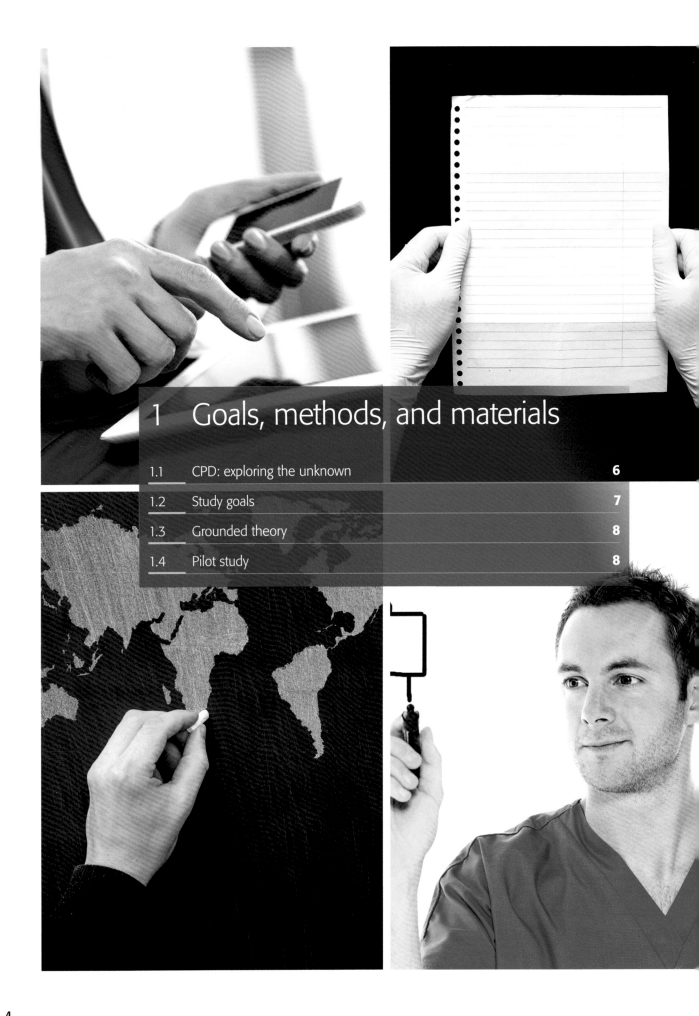

1 Goals, methods, and materials

1
Goals, methods, and materials

The educational needs and preferences of orthopedic and trauma surgeons at community hospitals have never been investigated. This group of surgeons treats the majority of trauma and orthopedic patients around the world. Examining the role of Continuing Professional Development (CPD) regulations and existing learning resources motivated this study.

Continuing Professional Development (CPD) for health professionals was introduced to improve the care given to patients. Effective CPD enhances the knowledge base of these individuals allowing the practice of new techniques and skills before they are applied in patient treatment. Improving CPD learning through better teaching would, therefore, be expected to result in fewer clinical errors being made.

Although there is a large body of evidence showing that CPD activities improve knowledge, skills and attitudes, resulting in improvements in patient care [1,2,3], the effect is often limited [4,5,6,7]. Understanding why this happens might lead to more effective education.

In 2009, the AO Foundation commissioned a study looking at the career pathways of orthopedic and trauma surgeons throughout the world. If career pathways of surgeons, and their changing educational needs and preferences, could be understood, then educational support for surgeons could be better organized, resulting in improved learning outcomes and better patient care. The study cumulated in the 2012 publication of a book: "Changing Patterns of Lifelong Learning": A study in surgeon education [8].

The study, which looked at the changing patterns of surgeon career pathways over time, also investigated the past, current and future educational needs of 147 surgeon interviewees. Participants were randomly selected for interview from a database of AO Foundation members. The results showed that surgeons who were currently actively involved with the AO organization were more likely to respond to the invitation than

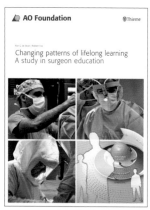

Complementary study

In the study "Changing patterns of lifelong learning", published by the AO in 2012, surgeons working outside large hospitals were underrepresented. The present study aims to correct this and should be seen as a complementary investigation.

those who had a looser or non-existent relationship. The results were bi-ased towards those surgeons who were already involved in teaching and learning. Although there was a good geographic spread of respondents, sur-geons working outside large hospitals were underrepresented in the data.

Globally, the majority of trauma and orthopedic patients are treated outside major teaching hospitals by surgeons who have no active role in teaching. For these reasons it was decided to investigate the learning needs and preferences of consultant staff working in community hospitals who had no relationship with a teaching organization.

1.1   CPD: exploring the unknown

Four aspects of Continued Professional Development (CPD) were of special interest and motivated the study.

- **Learning in a community hospital**
  Postgraduate medical education of health professionals is usually centered in large teaching hospitals, many of which have a university affiliation. On the other hand, most health care is delivered through smaller community hospitals where formal educational programs for staff are less structured. Information about how community hospitals organize their educational activities is limited and even less is known about how their staff respond to these activities.

- **Informal learning**
  Many studies have tried to identify the reasons for the success or failure of various education programs, but most studies have concentrated on the methods used [9,10]. In the past, education of health professionals has often focused on training events, the effectiveness of which is variable [11,12,13,14]. Internet-based activities have grown in recent years but have also had inconsistent success [15,16,17,18]. Little is known about the informal learning that occurs as part of everyday clinical activities, and whether it can be facilitated, despite the fact that this form of learning is the most common [19].

- **Cultural differences**
  Highly developed health care systems, such as those within the United States [20], have defined requirements for health professionals to maintain their professional status. This in turn has led to pressure from surgeons to ensure that they receive adequate education to retain their professional designation. Developing countries have very different systems of main-taining professional standards, varying from none to highly sophisticated ones. Very little is known about the requirements for postgraduate medical education outside the English-speaking world, and even less about the systems in place to meet this need [21].

- **Impact of CME regulations on community hospital doctors**
  Many countries have introduced systems to ensure that their doctors keep themselves up-to-date by attending approved educational events [22]. In some countries complex regulations exist requiring doctors to document their educational activities. Frequently this involves collecting a certain number of "CPD /CME points(continued professional development / continuing medical education) within a given timescale, typically 5 years. Anecdotally, the adherence of doctors to CPD regulations is inconsistent and systems may not function as they were designed to do. This study investigates the formal CPD requirements for doctors in different countries, where CPD exists, and compares this with the reality of practice. It also asks whether CPD requirements prompt doctors to look for education.

1.2   Study goals

The study proposal was submitted to the AO Education platform in 2011 and the following goals were agreed upon:

- Identify, by Internet search and personal interviews, those responsible for CPD. Identify the current programs for CPD for orthopedic and trauma surgeons working in community hospitals. Compare the data obtained by Internet search on CME/CPD requirements with the reality of existing programs and surgeon behavior.

- Explore the learning needs and preferences of postgraduate health professionals working in community hospitals and see whether existing programs and resources meet these needs and preferences.

- Uncover barriers that prevent health professionals from benefiting from CPD programs or being able to apply what they learned.

- Create a report identifying the different stages of postgraduate medical education that exist throughout the world.

- Produce a downloadable handbook for those responsible for education within a community hospital to advise on the most effective ways of educating their staff. The handbook would be freely available to all participants and to any hospital that wished to use it.

The pilot study phase involved interviewing surgeons from two countries (India and the United Kingdom). Their responses informed the creation of a standardized questionnaire that was then used in all of the subsequent interviews. Collection of country-specific continuing medical education requirements was also performed.

Designed to examine the educational needs and preferences of orthopedic and trauma surgeons working in community hospitals, the aim of this study was to explain a process and not to test or verify an existing theory; therefore, the grounded theory approach of Glaser and Strauss was used [23].

1.3   Grounded theory

Most orthopedic surgeons are familiar with research in which data is collected to support or refute a hypothesis. For example, a new implant is developed to meet a clinical need and the new implant is then rigorously tested to see if it satisfies the identified need. Grounded theory works in a different way. Data is collected without reference to a hypothesis. Once the data is collected analysis leads to a hypothesis based on the data. In this case, data was collected to see how surgeons working in community hospitals organize their education.

One goal of the method is to formulate hypotheses based on conceptual ideas. Another goal of a grounded theory study is to discover the participants' main concern and how they continually try to resolve it. The questions the researcher repeatedly asks in grounded theory are "What's going on?" and "What is the main problem of the participants, and "How are they trying to solve it?" Grounded theory studies are usually "qualitative" without using statistical methods. The results of a grounded theory study are not a set of statistically significant probabilities, but a set of probability statements about the relationship between concepts.

The question that may arise is: "How can a reader judge whether a given grounded theory study has validity?" Glaser suggests that a study should be judged by fit, relevance, workability, and modifiability [24].

- **Fit**
  How closely the theory generated corresponds to the incidents represented.
- **Relevance**
  A relevant study deals with the real concern of participants. It captures their attention and is not only of academic interest.
- **Workability**
  The theory works when it explains how the problem is being solved with much variation.
- **Modifiability**
  A modifiable theory can be altered when new relevant data is compared to existing data. A grounded theory is never right or wrong, it just has more or less fit, relevance, workability and modifiability.

1.4   Pilot study

In accordance with grounded theory's iterative study design, the pilot study involved interviewing 11 surgeons from two countries (India and the United Kingdom). These surgeons were then asked open-ended questions about their educational needs, preferences, resources and the barriers they faced in trying to keep themselves up-to-date. India and the UK were chosen to ensure that the pilot results reflected the diversity of responses that were expected from the study.

India does not have a robust continuing medical education (CME) system. Its medical services vary from highly developed tertiary care facilities to small hospitals with very limited resources. Doctors working in several small hospitals in a provincial town in Tamil Nardu were selected for interview.

The UK has a well established system of CPD and is beginning a re-accreditation process for consultant surgeons that involves, amongst other requirements, proof of involvement in CPD activities. Six surgeons from a community hospital in the northeast of England were interviewed. A single interviewer who had previously worked as a consultant orthopedic surgeon conducted the interviews.

In addition to the surgeons interviewed in the UK, the Chief Executive of the employing authority responsible for ensuring medical staff were adequately trained, was interviewed. No corresponding post existed in the Indian town included in the study.

None of the surgeons interviewed had any active relationship with the AO Foundation, but eight of the surgeons had attended an AO course when they were in training. None were or had been AO Faculty.

Prior to the interviews, details on relevant CPD requirements for doctors were gathered from the General Medical Council of Great Britain and the Tamil Nadu Medical Association. This information was obtained by accessing the relevant websites, and in the case of the United Kingdom, by a telephone call to an official.

Following analysis of the pilot data, the interview template was revised to reflect the themes of the pilot interviews. Analysis of pilot study data informed the design of the next cycle of data acquisition and an interview template was created for the main study (See page 41).

The main study involved a further eight sets of interviews that were carried out in eight different countries— Germany, Poland, Netherlands, Israel, China (PRC), Bangladesh, the Philippines and Thailand. An additional 39 surgeons were interviewed from 18 different hospitals, none of which was a major center.

As was the case with the pilot interviews, details on the relevant CPD regulations were obtained before the interviews took place. This information was researched online for Germany, United Kingdom. Poland, Netherlands. Israel, India, Bangladesh Philippines, Thailand. Information regarding China and the Philippines was obtained by interviews with local doctors.

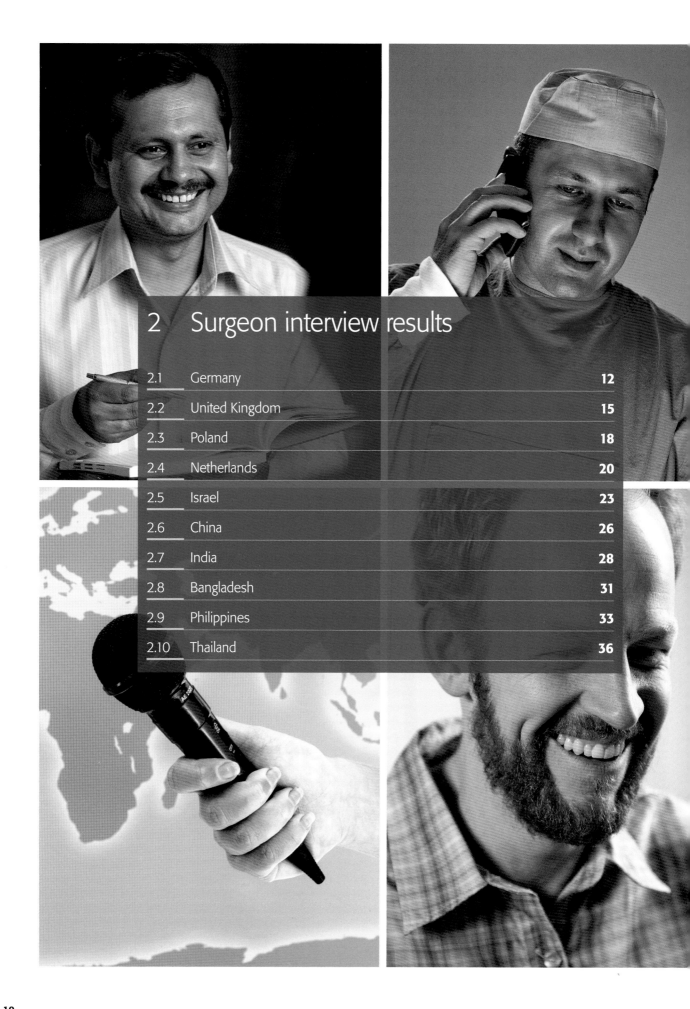

2 Surgeon interview results

2
Surgeon interview results

Orthopedic and trauma surgeons practicing in community hospitals were interviewed about their continuing education needs and preferences. Interviewees selected from ten countries shared varied experiences about their most beneficial learning opportunities and gave insight into their hopes for future education.

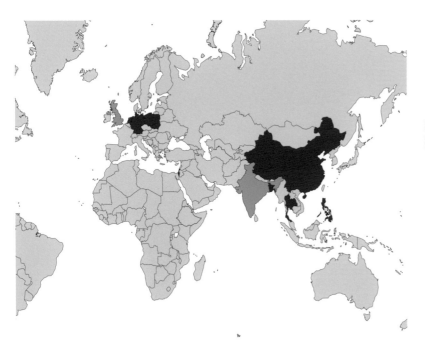

■ Pilot study
■ Added countries for main study

In the pilot study 11 surgeons from the United Kingdom and India were interviewed. The main study involved another set of interviews from Germany, United Kingdom, Poland, Netherlands, Israel, China, Bangladesh, Philippines, and Thailand (A total 39 surgeons from 18 different hospitals).

Using the interview template created from pilot study data, the project continued forward. When completied it involved 50 orthopedic surgeons who worked in community hospitals in 10 countries. Department size varied considerably: from surgeons who worked in solo practice to those working in departments that had more than eight qualified orthopedic specialists.

Of the ten countries represented, five were from the developed world: Germany, United Kingdom, Poland, Netherlands, Israel. Five were so called "developing countries": China, India, Bangladesh, Philippines, Thailand. This chapter summarizes the responses of surgeons, alphabetically by country, into the following categories. For a complete list of questions used during the study interview refer to page 41.

- Why surgeons look for education
- Importance of CPD accreditation
- Most recent search for CPD
- Changes in practice within the past year
- Top educational experience
- Printed material use
- Internet use for education
- Importance of courses, meetings and symposia
- Ease of informal discussions within units
- Importance of product related education
- Existing education facilities and barriers
- Suggestions for improving community hospital surgeon education

2.1 Germany

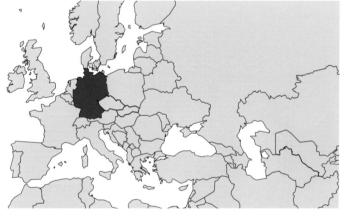

Number of surgeons interviewed

Five German surgeons with experience from 4 to 14 years post specialist training were interviewed. They came from 2 community hospitals, 1 private and 1 government operated. The government hospital had 6 specialists who served a population of 250,000. Their hospital was situated within 10 km of a large trauma unit. The private hospital had 5 specialists and served a population of 200,000. It carried out mainly elective trauma and orthopedic procedures. It was within 5 km of a major trauma unit. Neither hospital had surgical residents in training.

2.1.1 Why surgeons look for education
All five surgeons identified clinical problems as being either the most important or the only reason why they seek educational support. New technology was important to all, with one commenting that it was quite critical to his field and the main reason he looked for education. This surgeon had an interest in spinal surgery.

2.1.2 Importance of CPD accreditation
Collecting CPD accreditation points was not important to any surgeon. Two said that they needed to collect points because they were in private practice.

The other three said they collected points, but points were not vital to them. In the private system CPD accreditation does not exist, although there are plans to see if it can be introduced. For doctors who treat government patients there are strict CPD regulations but, in general terms, these consist of acquiring points to prove that the doctors are kept up-to-date through education. In Germany, CPD points are related to the number of hours of teaching and have nothing to do with quality or effectiveness.

2.1.3   Most recent search for CPD

The surgeons described elective orthopedic problems as the reason for their most recent search for education and identified a personal visit or an interaction with a colleague as being critical in helping to solve the problem. Two of the surgeons had initially looked for solutions using books and online material but in the end had to contact a colleague.

2.1.4   Changes in practice within the past year

Each of the surgeons had changed at least one aspect of their practice in the last year. All modifications were related to a change in instrumentation. In two cases, the resources used to bring about change were discussions with an expert. One surgeon made the change after participating in a short-term fellowship. One surgeon changed his practice following discussions with a company representative and two attended workshops, one of which was commercially sponsored.

2.1.5   Top educational experience

All five surgeons identified discussions with experts and friends as their best ever learning experience. One commented that these discussions now usually took place online rather than by phone or personal contact.

2.1.6   Printed material use

Classic textbooks were referenced by all interviewees. Three surgeons described their use of books as a way to refresh their memory. They felt that books were most useful when you thought you knew what you were doing and the books confirmed it. One surgeon commented that he was able to access certain information faster using the books he already knew than going online via a search engine.

None of the five surgeons read journals on a regular basis. All looked to journals from time to time but one surgeon commented that he had no time to read full articles. When the surgeons wanted instant information, they went online to look for evidence supporting their decision making.

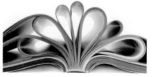

Journals rarely read

None of the five surgeons from Germany read journals on a regular basis. When they wanted instant information, they went online.

2.1.7   Internet use for education

The Internet was identified as being the major source for information, particularly in regard to new technology. Three of the surgeons used Pub Med as a search engine. None of the surgeons used a professional website.

When it came to describing their ideal website, three of the surgeons said that they would like to have the ability to contact experts and to tap into a network of experience. The other two surgeons said they wanted access to a website where relevant information had already been sorted for them. They wished to have selected articles made available without having to use a search engine.

2.1.8   Importance of courses, meetings and symposia

Large national meetings were attended by all interviewees. Two surgeons attended meetings related to their own orthopedic subspecialty. The other three attended larger meetings such as those orgenaized by the American Academy of Orthopedic Surgeons (AAOS). All five felt that speaking with friends and colleagues at these meetings was the main reason for going.

None of the surgeons had regular hospital meetings, although all held ward and business rounds.

2.1.9   Ease of informal discussions within units

Four surgeons commented that they had difficulty contacting their colleagues while working in the hospital. Being busy and little time were identified as the limiting factors. The fifth surgeon described poor interpersonal relationships within his hospital.

2.1.10   Importance of product related education

New product information provided by representatives of commercial companies was accessed by all five surgeons. Two surgeons specifically stated that they refused to see company representatives who called at their hospitals or requested an appointment. However, company representatives would be called on if the surgeon wanted access to specific new technology.

Two surgeons had attended training events on how to be a better teacher. For one surgeon it was part of his university training. The second had attended an "AO Tips for Trainers Course". Those who had training to be better teachers felt the experience was important to their clinical practice and teaching.

2.1.11   Existing education facilities and barriers

Internet access was identified as the only resource for education provided by the hospital. Three of the surgeons had no difficulty accessing education outside the hospital. A fourth said the issue was time; he commented, "When I am not working I am not earning."

None of the surgeons felt that the hospital had a responsibility for their education. One said that he would appreciate faster Internet connection.

2.1.12   Suggestions for improving community hospital surgeon education

A desire for some form of Internet community was expressed by four of the five surgeons. They described this as access to a network of excellence. There was a concern as to who could join such a network and who the experts were. The fifth surgeon commented that he would like short educational courses based on the needs of his patients.

2.2   United Kingdom

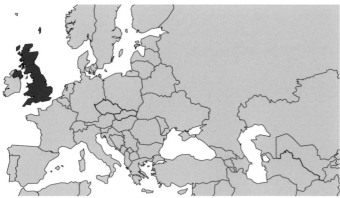

†††††††
Number of surgeons interviewed

Of the 6 surgeons interviewed, experience ranged considerably—from 2 to 30 years since completion of specialist orthopedic training. All UK interviewees were from a single community hospital that serves a population of 150,000 people. The nearest larger hospital was 60 km away where the orthopedic unit employed 11 specialists.

2.2.1   Why surgeons look for education

All six surgeons agreed that clinical problems were usually the motivation for seeking educational help. Four surgeons felt that because they worked in relatively small units, new technology was not an important driver of education for them. However, two of the surgeons disagreed and felt new technology was a common reason for them to look for education.

2.2.2   Importance of CPD accreditation

Of the six surgeons interviewed, two felt that CPD accreditation points were very important when assessing education opportunities. One stated that CPD accreditation points were "a must have" and he would go to an event merely to pick up the points. Three surgeons felt that CPD accreditation was not important in any significant way, and the remaining surgeon said that although he knew he should collect points, he did not know how to.

2.2.3   Most recent search for continuing medical education

Two interviewees reported that an acute trauma problem was the reason they last sought education; the others wanted help with orthopedic problems. The resources that they accessed to resolve these problems were variable. Three of the surgeons used the Internet as their source of information, and one of these surgeons subsequently had a discussion with a friend. Four of the surgeons felt discussions with colleagues were a major educational asset.

2.2.4   Changes in practice within the past year

Changes in practice had been made by five of the surgeons within the past year. Only one of these changes related to trauma. Two of the surgeons used the Internet as their main educational tool to make the change, two respondents attended courses run by implant manufacturers, and one surgeon said that hospital management had imposed the changes he made.

2.2.5   Top educational experience

Although the interviewees had considerable variability with regards to the educational resources that they used in everyday practice, five surgeons said their best educational experience involved interpersonal relationships with colleagues. Four of the surgeons were unable to form these relationships within their own unit and used colleagues from other units to discuss problem cases. One surgeon felt that the presence of a new colleague had radically altered his practice for the better as he now had someone to talk to within his unit. The remaining surgeon felt that his best educational experience was a workshop during a course.

2.2.6   Printed material use

Books were used by three of the surgeons as educational aids to refamiliarize themselves with something or to refresh their memory. The use of books was not related to the seniority of the surgeons.

Five surgeons read print journals, not electronic versions, on a regular basis. They only looked at articles that were relevant to their particular practice.

2.2.7   Internet use for education

The Internet was used a lot by five interviewees to gather information. In this particular hospital, management had required all surgeons to take eLearning modules related to child protection. The surgeons did not regard this eLearning module as being relevant to their needs and were very hostile to the idea of eLearning as being part of an educational portfolio.

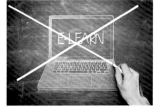

Crossing out eLearning
The UK hospital management had required all the surgeons to take eLearning modules related to child protection. They did not regard this eLearning module as being relevant.

In terms of preferred search engine, Google was used by four and the other two had no preferences. Three of the surgeons had preferred professional websites which included: the AO Surgery Reference, Wheeless and ShoulderDoc, as well as doctor.net.

Perhaps because of the negative experience regarding the compulsory eLearning module none of the surgeons were keen on further development of web-based education, apart from one who said that it would be useful to gain access to research articles for free.

2.2.8   Importance of courses, meetings and symposia

Five of the surgeons attended large national educational events. Three attended the British Orthopaedic Association annual meeting, one attended the annual meeting of a specialist society, and the fifth attended the Edinburgh Trauma Course. They felt that interaction with colleagues was the most important thing when attending an event. One surgeon attended annual meetings merely to pick up CPD points. The surgeons go to these events to keep themselves up-to-date, with the exception of one surgeon who was faculty on a hip replacement course.

Hospital meetings were held every day: these were largely administrative and not educational. Every six weeks there was an audit meeting described as having become a management meeting rather than a clinical one.

2.2.9   Ease of informal discussions within units

Carrying out informal discussions within their hospital was difficult for all six surgeons. Two issues were outlined: the first was that it was very difficult to find the time to talk to individuals. Agendas were full and there was no space in them for scheduling a meeting. If one surgeon had time his colleague would often be busy and unavailable. The second issue, which affected four of the six surgeons, was that they felt there was nobody within their own unit to have useful conversations with. All the surgeons had developed specialist interests and these four surgeons did not have a colleague colleague to talk about cases that fell within their field of expertise.

2.2.10   Importance of product related education

Education offered by commercial companies was useful to four surgeons. They felt it was a good way of keeping up-to-date with new technology. They also appreciated workshops carried out by the companies. All the surgeons were aware of commercial bias but felt that they were able to deal with this when discussing new technologies.

One surgeon had received training to be a teacher and he was an Advanced Trauma Life Support (ATLS) instructor.

2.2.11   Existing education facilities and barriers

The doctors identified no significant educational resources within the hospital. Getting leave was the major barrier to accessing education for all of them. There were two issues with regard to this. Firstly, they commented that working in a small unit meant that a minimum number of consultants had to be left within the hospital to cover any situation. The second point was they felt pressured by management to push through cases rather than access education. Given this, it makes sense that five of the six surgeons wanted their hospital to give them protected leave to help with their education.

2.2.12   Suggestions for improving community hospital surgeon education

Two surgeons mentioned having experts available to discuss difficult cases, either through hospital visits or online contact. A third one said that he would like the ability to refer complex cases he felt he could not handle.

Due to the relatively small unit size, there was an overall sense of providing basic services for the community and feeling rather isolated. The unit size and lack of specialist expertise within the local consultant community led to unique educational problems.

2.3   Poland

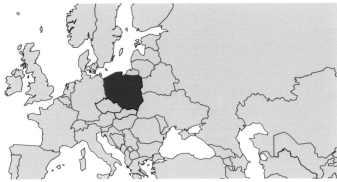

Number of surgeons interviewed

The 5 Polish surgeons who were interviewed hailed from 3 different community hospitals, which served populations between 150,000 and 300,000 people. The experience of the surgeons ranged from 4 to 15 years post specialist registration. The unit size varied from 4 to 8 specialist orthopedic surgeons.

2.3.1   Why surgeons look for education
Clinical problems were the motivation for seeking education for all the surgeons. One surgeon felt that new technology was a very important driver for him, but the other four said that new technology was difficult to introduce into their hospitals and was therefore not so important.

2.3.2   Importance of CPD accreditation
Regulations and collection of points were completely unimportant to all interviewees. They reported that a CPD accreditation system did exist within Poland but there was disagreement about who should run it. The system had fallen into disrepute, and as a result was ignored by most surgeons.

2.3.3   Most recent search for CPD
Trauma cases were identified by all five surgeons as being the most recent reason they looked for education. Three of the five solved their problems by interaction with a colleague. Two of these discussions were carried out online after sending CTs and other information to a trusted friend. One clinical problem was resolved after discussing it with a senior surgeon from the same hospital. The other two surgeons used books to solve their clinical problems.

2.3.4   Changes in practice within the past year
All five surgeons had introduced new technology, and in particular changes to trauma instrumentation, in the past year.

Information supplied by implant manufacturers was employed by four surgeons to affect the changes—a combination of visits from company representatives and commercial website videos were used. The fifth surgeon brought about change by attending a non-commercial seminar, which had practical workshops sponsored by an implant manufacturer. Although all the surgeons accepted that commercial bias was inevitable with the material supplied by implant manufacturers, they felt this did not influence their decision whether or not to introduce new technology.

2.3.5   Top educational experience

An interaction with another surgeon was reported as the best educational experience by all interviewees. One of the surgeons achieved this through a fellowship, another by attending an AO course. The others described relationships that formed during their training or in the early part of their independent practice. All these interactions centred on a clinical problem or a single case.

2.3.6   Printed material use

Books were regularly used by four surgeons; however, the fifth stated he had no time to read books. "Standard texts", which were often quite old, were used as a reference, and it was mentioned that they knew where to find the answers within their books.

Journals were rarely used by the five surgeons. This was for a variety of reasons: the lack of journal articles published in Polish was a major problem for three of them, and getting access to full articles seemed also to be a problem.

2.3.7   Internet use for education

All five surgeons extensively used the Internet to do research. One commented it was his first port of call when faced with a clinical problem; however, it was difficult to access websites published in Polish.

In terms of search engines, two of the surgeons used "PubMed", one used Google, and one used "Medline". Two surgeons used the website of the American Academy of Orthopedic Surgeons (AAOS) as their preferred specialist site.

Availability of more video-based online material was desired by three of the five surgeons, especially videos made by experienced surgeons showing surgical approaches, real surgery and above all, tips and tricks. However, one surgeon was very negative about the Internet saying that eLearning only works if what was being taught was relevant to your problem.

2.3.8   Importance of courses, meetings and symposia

Large annual congresses were attended by all five, with a preference for meetings covering a large range of topics. All the surgeons faced major difficulties attending courses. The three that attended courses felt the opportunity to talk to their colleagues was the most important reason for attendance. However, two major barriers were identified: for those working in smaller units, it was difficult to arrange leave, and financial constraints prevented attendance unless sponsorship from an industrial partner was received.

Daily trauma rounds in their hospitals were the norm for all the surgeons, but these were considered administrative and not educational. One surgeon, who had juniors within his hospital, had a monthly journal club. Four surgeons had monthly visits from commercial companies that sponsored academic meetings in exchange for getting time to present new products to the surgeons.

2.3.9   Ease of informal discussions within units

Informal discussions within their hospitals were difficult for three of the five surgeons. The difficulties centred on interpersonal issues with senior colleagues. However, these three – who had graduated from the same teaching institute,

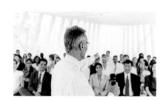

Difficulties attending courses

All six Polish surgeons had major difficulties attending courses. For those working in smaller units it was challenging to arrange leave. Additionally, financial constraints prevents attendance unless industry sponsorship was received.

had set up an online group they could interact with. The fourth surgeon said that usually there was no problem with informal discussions in his hospital, but if no one knew the answer he would try to find someone elsewhere that he knew he could trust. One surgeon said that although there were no problems it would be nice if these meetings could be put on a more formal basis.

2.3.10 Importance of product related education
Four surgeons found that commercial companies provided very important information, particularly in regard to new technology. The importance of company sponsorship for education within their hospitals was acknowledged by three interviewees. One surgeon felt, however, that the impact of this type of information was minimal. All surgeons reported that they were aware of commercial bias in the material provided by companies but they felt the bias did not significantly influence their clinical decision making.

2.3.11 Existing education facilities and barriers
Four of the five surgeons had no educational resources within their hospital, while the fifth had a very useful library. Major barriers with regards to accessing educational events, especially courses, were identified by all respondents. Although time was an issue for two surgeons, financial constraints were more important and were mentioned by all the surgeons.

2.3.12 Suggestions for improving community hospital surgeon education
Four surgeons commented that the standards within their hospital varied from surgeon to surgeon and they felt that the hospital should introduce minimum standards of care. All five surgeons felt that there was a role for government and hospitals to annually review minimum education standards for doctors. All the surgeons interviewed felt that there were significant numbers of surgeons practicing suboptimal medicine.

2.4   Netherlands

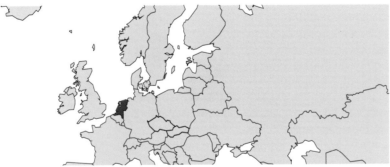

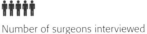
Number of surgeons interviewed

In the Netherlands, the 5 surgeons who were interviewed worked in 2 different community hospitals that were linked by a single management team. Surgical experience of the interviewees varied between 5 and 26 years from completion of specialist orthopedic training. The nearest large hospital with a specialized trauma unit was 40 km away.

2.4.1   Why surgeons look for education

All the surgeons interviewed agreed that clinical problems led them to look for educational support. This was most likely when unfamiliar clinical problems were encountered or when something had gone wrong. New technology was also a driver of education but only one of the five surgeons felt that it was very important. He was particularly interested in new advances in arthroplasty.

2.3.2   Importance of CPD accreditation

CPD points for re-accreditation were required of all the surgeons and points were easily collected. All five surgeons said that CPD accreditation of an event was not important when deciding which educational events to attend.

2.4.3   Most recent search for CPD

Trauma problems were identified by all five surgeons as being the most recent reason for seeking educational support. All the surgeons dealt with their last problem by talking to a colleague. Three of the five did this face-to-face, the other two sent x-rays to a colleague via the Internet.

2.4.4   Changes in practice within the past year

Changes to the orthopedic practices of all the surgeons had occurred in the last year, all related to elective orthopedic surgery.

Two of the surgeons said that they had made this change as a result of attending a course. They identified the course's practical elements as being the most important to them. The other three had initiated change after discussions with a colleague.

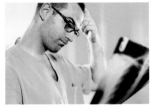

Educational support needed
Trauma problems were identified by all five Dutch surgeons as being the most recent reason for seeking educational support. The surgeons dealt with their last problem either by talking to a colleague or sending x-rays.

2.4.5   Top educational experience

All the surgeons identified personal interactions as being the key to their best educational experiences. Three surgeons reported that this occurred during their surgical training. All three described being guided through the operative management of a patient by a senior surgeon. The other two achieved this when attending an innovative course that featured workshops and the ability to discuss clinical problems with faculty.

2.4.6   Printed material use

Three of the surgeons still used books extensively, primarily to refresh their memory. Classic textbooks, especially anatomy books, were important to them. One surgeon commented that looking at his old books was a faster way of getting relevant information than using the Internet because he knew exactly where to look.

None of the surgeons used journals extensively. Only one subscribed to a journal on a personal basis and he said that he rarely read the articles. Two respondents accessed journal articles through an Internet search engine

2.4.7   Internet use for education

The Internet was used by all of the respondents as a way of getting factual information, as well as for communication. The Dutch surgeons used a variety of search engines including: Google, PubMed and Medline. They did not identify any professional websites they used on a regular basis.

Three of the surgeons expressed the desire to get practical advice via the Internet. They wanted the ability to ask questions and get answers but there were issues: none of the three wanted an open access website where anyone could post cases or make a comment. One surgeon remarked: "I only want advice from people I trust." In addition, two of the surgeons wished to have access to videos online. They were particularly keen to see videos about surgical techniques. For maximum educational effect the videos should include commentary.

2.4.8   Importance of courses, meetings and symposia
One big annual national meeting was attended by all the surgeons; four of the five felt that attending a big meeting was a good way to keep up-to-date and catch up with old friends. They saw it as a chance to learn about new clinical advances and find out what was happening professionally and socially with their friends and colleagues from other units. The fifth surgeon attended an annual meeting but was not happy with the education he got there.

All the surgeons attended hospital meetings on a regular basis. Two of the surgeons had junior surgeons in their hospital who were still in training and these sessions were felt to be very important not only for teaching but also learning.

2.4.9   Ease of informal discussions within units
No surgeon reported any difficulty in interacting with colleagues. They all felt that they worked together as a team. Although all the surgeons were busy and worked at two sites they felt there was usually time during the day for discussion.

2.4.10   Importance of product related education
Good, nonbiased relationships between commercial company representatives and surgeons were reported by all. It was universally commented that there were very tight regulatory arrangements within the Netherlands to ensure that these relationships remained ethically acceptable. All surgeons felt that contact with company representatives was an extremely good way of keeping up-to-date with technological advances, and two said it was the most important way of doing so.

One of the surgeons was an Advanced Trauma Life Instructor (ATLS) and had attended a faculty development event. He felt that his training as a teacher had helped him enormously in his clinical practice.

2.4.11   Existing education facilities and barriers
In terms of existing hospital resources, three of the surgeons had access to the Internet and a library within the hospital, while the other two had no significant educational resources within their hospital. The library was not felt to be useful for the surgeons interviewed, but was a useful resource for the surgeons in training.

With regards to attending educational events, one of the surgeons felt that he had no barriers, while the other three said there was occasional difficulty in getting leave because of the size of their unit. They commented that with adequate planning attendance at an educational event was usually possible.

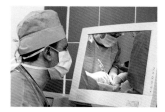

Learning with video

Two of the five surgeons from the Netherlands wished to have access to videos online. They were particularly keen to get videos about surgical techniques with commentary.

2.4.12   Suggestions for improving community hospital surgeon education

Although their hospitals were generally supportive, three of the surgeons felt that management did not understand that doctors needed to continually refresh their skills throughout their career. They felt that if hospital management better understood this issue it would help.

Two of the surgeons said that refresher courses specifically targeted to senior surgeons would be very attractive to them. They also said that these courses should be highly interactive and relatively short. The other three surgeons felt that the most important thing for them was the opportunity to discuss cases with others, including surgeons working in different units. There were no clear ideas about how this might be achieved apart from using the possibilities of the Internet.

2.5   Israel

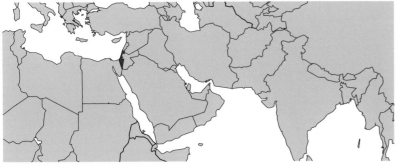

Number of surgeons interviewed

Four Israeli surgeons with experience ranging from 7 to 23 years post specialist registration were interviewed. The surgeons came from 3 different government-owned community hospitals serving populations between 100,000 and 200,000 people. One of the hospitals had close links with a major teaching hospital and had residents in training; all were situated within 40 km of a major trauma unit.

2.5.1   Why surgeons look for education

Clinical issues were usually the reason that all the Israeli surgeons sought educational help. All four used new technology, but just one of the surgeons felt that this constituted a significant reason to look for education.

2.4.2   Importance of CPD accreditation

None of the surgeons interviewed felt that CPD was important to them in any way. They reported that there is no formal CPD accreditation process within Israel. Consultants are not required to undertake any period of formal education during their working day/week. There is no system for continual evaluation of consultants, appraisal, or assessment. There are no proposals to introduce such a system. It follows, therefore, that CPD accreditation is totally unimportant to all Israeli consultants.

2.5.3   Most recent search for CPD

Recent complex orthopedic problems spurred three surgeons to seek education, while the fourth surgeon stated that he looked for educational help to ensure his general standards of practice were up-to-date.

Professional interactions were mentioned by all four surgeons as a help in resolving their most recent clinical problems. Two of these interactions were carried out with colleagues at the hospital. The third was carried out with a colleague at a second hospital. The fourth surgeon had taken the opportunity to discuss a specific clinical issue with a number of surgeons while attending an educational course.

2.5.4   Changes in practice within the past year

All four surgeons had changed at least one aspect of their clinical practice in the last year, with three surgeons altering an aspect of their orthopedic practice and one changing an aspect of his trauma practice. All four surgeons used some form of discussion to affect the change. Two of the changes occurred as a result of discussions with colleagues, and two happened after discussion with representatives of medical device companies.

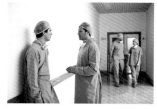

Discussing change

All four Israeli surgeons questioned used some form of discussion to affect change. Two of the changes occurred as a result of discussions with colleagues, and two happened after discussion with representatives of medical device companies.

2.5.5   Top educational experience

Interactions such as working with people and experts, were by far the best education experience for all the interviewees. One of the experiences described was a result of a formal fellowship, the other three occasions were informal and consisted of working with a colleague who had expertise and doing a case together.

2.5.6   Printed material use

Only half of the surgeons used books in any way. Both of them recognized their books were getting out of date and tended to use them to confirm that their actions were correct rather than to find out new information.

Due to the time needed to read journals, three of the four surgeons did not read them. The fourth surgeon, however, browsed his copy of "The Journal of Bone & Joint Surgery" every month.

2.5.7   Internet use for education

Internet use was prevalent with all four surgeons, who agreed that it was the best educational resource when looking for information. One of the surgeons particularly liked looking at videos of surgical procedures. Three of the surgeons used Google as their search engine and the other used PubMed.

Two websites were regularly visited by half of the respondents: American Academy of Orthopaedic Surgeons and www.trauma.org.

None of the surgeons advocated eLearning as a way forward for their own education. None of them suggested a way in which the Internet could become friendlier for them. One surgeon commented that he had been forced to do a 30-hour online course on evidence-based medicine as part of his training and he hated it.

2.5.8   Importance of courses, meetings and symposia

A large annual meeting was attended by three of the four surgeons. Those three surgeons felt that the ability to speak with friends and colleagues was the reason they went there. In regard to meetings, they prefer those, were many topics are under discussion so they can pick and choose what to attend.

All four surgeons had daily meetings connected with trauma in their hospital. Physiotherapists also attended the meetings. All four surgeons felt that these daily ward rounds were a great way of learning, as well as teaching some of the juniors.

2.5.9   Ease of informal discussions within units
The most experienced surgeon felt isolated within his unit because he was the senior person and there was nobody with sufficient expertise for him to talk to. The remaining three surgeons reported no difficulty in having informal discussions in their workplace.

2.5.10   Importance of product related education
Extremely positive responses were received regarding the impact of education from commercial companies. All four surgeons said that contact with the company representatives was a great way of keeping up-to-date. They also liked the commercial websites that were available, particularly the videos there, and used them frequently. They were aware of commercial bias in the material that they had been given, but felt that they did not allow this to influence their clinical decision making.

None of the surgeons had attended any form of faculty development event.

2.5.11   Existing education facilities and barriers
No significant educational resources within the hospitals were reported, apart from the presence of the daily trauma meeting.

None of the surgeons, all of whom were working in government service, had difficulty in accessing educational events due to time constraints or finances.

2.5.12   Suggestions for improving community hospital surgeon education
Three of the four surgeons said that their hospitals could help by giving them sufficient time to pursue independent learning during the day. Getting time off to attend an event was not problematic, but getting the time to access educational resources during clinical work proved to be difficult.

When asked about the one thing they would like to do to improve their own education, three surgeons answered "Speaking and interacting with other surgeons." Only one surgeon suggested how this could be done, which was to physically visit another hospital. Improving their interaction with colleagues and senior surgeons seems to be the most important request from this group of surgeons.

2.6   China

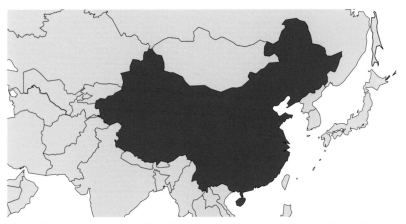

Five Chinese surgeons working in 2 community hospitals were interviewed. One hospital served a population of 2 million but it was not the local trauma center. The other hospital served a community of 750,000. Both units had 8 specialist orthopedic surgeons and both units had resident medical staff in training. Interviewee experience varied from 3 to 14 years from completion of specialist training.

Number of surgeons interviewed

2.6.1   Why surgeons look for education
All five surgeons agreed that clinical problems were the major reason why they looked for education on a day-to-day basis. They also described their most recent educational experience as being related to trauma. One surgeon commented that when confronted with a clinical problem he reads about it in the evening at home using a book.

2.6.2   Importance of CPD accreditation
Four of the surgeons interviewed were unaware of any CPD regulations applying to them. The fourth said that he was required to do 25 hours per year but because his hospital organized meetings this was something that he did not have to worry about.

2.6.3   Most recent search for CPD
Four surgeons dealt with their most recent clinical problem by getting advice from a colleague. In addition, two of them used books and the other two watched a video on the Internet.

2.6.4   Changes in practice within the past year
In the last year a change in practice had been made by three of the five surgeons. For these surgeons the change involved adopting minimally invasive surgery techniques using locking plates. The three who had made the change got the information by either speaking with colleagues or attending a workshop run by a company.

2.6.5   Top educational experience
Four of the five surgeons claimed that discussion with other doctors was their best educational experience, seeing what they were doing and speaking with

them. All had achieved this by attending national meetings. The fifth doctor felt that attendance at a cadaveric workshop with hands-on experience was his best ever educational experience.

2.6.6   Printed material use

Books were incredibly important to all five surgeons. Four commented that this may be due to their past educational experience. In China, books are an essential part of education from the age of five. All surgeons used standard textbooks that had been translated into Mandarin and felt that these books would never really be out-of-date because they contain principles. One stated the books are always very important because they were written by famous specialists who knew everything.

All five doctors used journals. They selectively read either the"Journal of Bone & Joint Surgery" or a specialist journal related to their interests.

2.6.7   Internet use for education

All five surgeons encountered major difficulties using the Internet. In fact, two did not bother to use it at all. The problems were slow data transfer and download times, which meant it was difficult to access information and almost impossible to watch videos. Much of what is online is not translated into Mandarin, which is a major issue. Finally, the Chinese government has banned Google which makes search more difficult. One of the surgeons said he used a search engine called Baidu. None of the surgeons accessed an academic website on a regular basis.

When it came to expressing what they wanted from the Internet all five basically wanted a faster Internet service. Their responses were concerned with the mechanics of the Internet and not the content. Access to articles in Chinese was very important for three of the five surgeons.

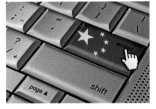

Internet access difficult
Major difficulties were encountered by all five Chinese surgeons while using the Internet. The problems were very slow download speeds, which meant it was very difficult to see videos and much of what is online is not translated into Mandarin.

2.6.8   Importance of courses, meetings and symposia

Educational events were attended by all five surgeons. Three of them said that national meetings were the most important because they provided an opportunity to speak to friends and colleagues. All five commented that that company provided courses were available more or less on a weekly basis, but most of them were of limited value.

All five surgeons had hospital meetings. Three worked in hospitals where there were visiting lecturers. Although lectures have been useful from the point of view of accumulating CME points the overall sense was that there was little value in them. Trauma rounds were present in one of the hospitals. No multidisciplinary meetings were attended by any of the surgeons.

2.6.9   Ease of informal discussions within units

Four of the five surgeons declared they had difficulties getting access to colleagues in their own hospital to discuss clinical issues. The fifth said it was easy to access his chiefs, but very difficult to get them to change their mind. Two surgeons used national meetings as a way of interacting with their colleagues.

2.6.10   Importance of product related education

All five surgeons had regular visits from pharmaceutical and medical device representatives. Everyone said that this was a very good way to get access to new products. Sponsorship of educational meetings was very important so that doctors in China who are poorly paid can attend.

2.6.11   Existing education facilities and barriers

No surgeon interviewed had received any instruction with regard to improving teaching skills.

All five surgeons reported very poor libraries in their hospital that were hardly used. Two have access to the Internet, but it is so slow it is virtually useless. Only one of the surgeons had difficulty accessing education because getting a leave of absence proved almost impossible. However, all five surgeons commented that if they did attend an educational event it was difficult to apply the technology because Chinese patients are expected to pay for their implants, and usually cannot afford new technologiy.

2.6.12   Suggestions for improving community hospital surgeon education

Interviewees felt that it was important for Chinese surgeons to be able to visit other countries and to have more opportunities to visit other centers within China. They felt that this was a responsibility of the government hospital service. It was summed up by one surgeon who stated: "We will not be able to provide the best service if we do not have access to new technology and experience."

2.7   India

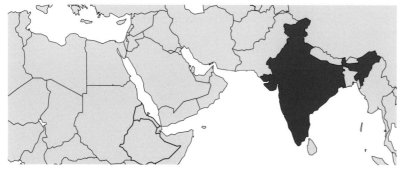

Number of surgeons interviewed

From a city of 3.5 million people, 5 Indian surgeons working in 4 small peripheral hospitals were interviewed. Three hospitals were private and 1 was run by the local government. Surgeon experience varied from 2 to 30 years post specialist registration. The size of orthopedic departments varied from 1 to 6 specialists, with 3 of the 5 surgeons having appointments in more than 1 hospital. The government hospital was the only one where residents in training were present.

2.7.1   Why surgeons look for education

The Indian surgeons stated "clinical problems" as the main reason education was accessed on a day-to-day basis. All five surgeons expressed interest in new techniques, and two of them focused on new technologies is an important reason for seeking education. However, the costs of new technologies and associated difficulties with funding made surgeons cautious about using them. Funding in a government hospital is severely limited in India and private patients have to pay for their implants.

2.7.2   Importance of CPD accreditation

Only one of the surgeons recognized CPD accreditation as being important to him in any way. He stated that there were no national requirements but the local State Medical Association had set up its own informal system of accrediting certain educational events. However, two of the surgeons commented that imposing some sort of CPD regulation would be important to improve clinical standards. They felt that doctors should be compelled to keep themselves up-to-date and this might best be achieved within a CPD framework.

2.7.3   Most recent search for CPD

All five surgeons cited clinical problems as the reason for their most recent access to education. All the cases involved fractures. This follows the pattern seen in other developing countries where trauma is often more important than elective orthopedics, both in government and private practice. To solve their problems three surgeons used books as their educational resource and the other two had a discussion with a colleague.

2.7.4   Changes in practice within the past year

Changes in practice had been incorporated by all five surgeons within the past year. All the changes related to the treatment of trauma patients and the introduction of new technologies. Working closely with a colleague was felt to be instrumental by three of the surgeons to achive change. One of these took a fellowship. The remaining two attended courses at a cadaver workshop where they collaborated closely with a senior surgeon The other two surgeons had received printed information from a representative of a medical device manufacturer.

2.7.5   Top educational experience

Interpersonal contact with other doctors was the key behind all five surgeons' most successful educational experiences. These included: being taken through a case by a colleague, and attending a fellowship. The third surgeon developed connections within his own personal network and the other two identified working closely with an expert at a workshop as being their best educational experience.

2.7.6   Printed material use

Four of the five surgeons said that books were their most important educational resource, citing a classic orthopedic textbook—Campbell's. One said he rarely used books.

All five surgeons read journals. Three subscribed to the "Journal of Bone & Joint Surgery" and they read every issue from cover to cover. The other two saw themselves as occasional readers.

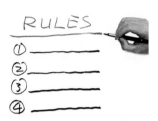

Obligation to learn

Two of the surgeons commented that one of the most important things that could be done to improve clinical standards would be to impose some form of CPD regulation.

2.7.7   Internet use for education

Two surgeons reported they used the Internet extensively to solve clinical problems. The remaining three did not use the Internet because of difficulties accessing the technology. Google was the only search engine mentioned and the AO Surgery Reference was the only professional website identified by any of the surgeons.

When it came to answering the question, "What do you want from the Internet?", two surgeons wished to have an Internet that worked, and one surgeon felt that he did not want any service available on the Internet. A fourth surgeon said that he wanted to be able to read entire articles, not just abstracts, and the fifth surgeon said that although he was happy to use the Internet to gain information he did not like using the Internet because it did not give him the personal interaction he wanted.

2.7.8   Importance of courses, meetings and symposia

Local state and regional congresses were attended by four surgeons; the fifth was unable to get sufficient leave of absence to attend these events. The three who did attend state meetings felt that discussing cases with friends and colleagues was a very important element. Two said that it was a major social event in their calendar. These surgeons would usually take their families to such a meeting.

Only one of the surgeons attended daily meetings in his hospital. The surgeon who had daily rounds felt that these were largely useless from an educational point of view.

2.7.9   Ease of informal discussions within units

Contact with other surgeons was identified as being very important to all interviewees. However, all five surgeons also commented that this was extremely difficult to organize in their hospitals due to the small size of the units. Four of the five wished to be able to discuss clinical problems with surgeons from other hospitals.

2.7.10   Importance of product related education

All of the surgeons had regular visits from sales people representing pharmaceutical and medical device companies. Only one felt that the visits were useful and the other four commented the only benefit was a free lunch.

2.7.11   Existing education facilities and barriers

One of the surgeons is an ATLS (Advanced Trauma Life Support) instructor. He felt that learning how to be a better teacher was very useful in all aspects of his clinical work.

All of the surgeons had very limited hospital resources to assist education. Two had no resources at all, and the other two had poor libraries together with slow Internet.

Three of the surgeons had problems attending educational events because leave of absence was difficult to obtain. This, again, was related to the size of the hospital.

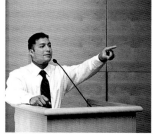

To be a better teacher

One of the surgeons is an ATLS (Advanced Trauma Life Support) instructor. He felt that learning how to be a better teacher was very useful in all aspects of his clinical work.

2.7.12   Suggestions for improving community hospital surgeon education
The need for hospitals to recognize the importance of medical education for their staff was articulated by three of the surgeons. They expressed a desire for more time to organize meetings, discuss cases, and listen to outside speakers. Three surgeons commented that there were no minimum standards of education education in India and they perceived a need for an external body to set standards. They also felt that although they accessed education if they encountered clinical problems, many of their colleagues practicing in the same city did not do so.

2.8   Bangladesh

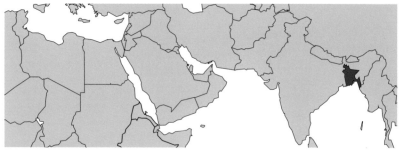

Number of surgeons interviewed

Five orthopedic surgeons varying in experience from 4 to 11 years post specialist registration were interviewed. They came from three hospitals, all of which were run by the government. The population served was approximately 3 million. 2 of the 3 hospitals had residents in training while the largest hospital had 18 specialists, the smallest, 6.

2.8.1   Why surgeons look for education
All surgeons interviewed felt that clinical problems were the main reason they accessed education. The vast majority of these problems were related to the management of trauma cases. All five surgeons were interested in new technology, but it was not their major motivation, largely because it is very difficult to introduce new technology in a poor country. Funding for implants is not readily available from the government and the patient usually must bear the cost of implants. Most patients and their families cannot afford to buy new implants.

2.8.2   Importance of CPD accreditation
None of the surgeons recognized CPD accreditation as being important to them in any way, and two were unaware of any CPD regulations applying to Bangladesh.

2.8.3   Most recent search for CPD
All five surgeons cited clinical problems as the reason they recently accessed education. All clinical problems were related to fracture cases. In Bangladesh, trauma is more important than orthopedics both in the public and private sector. Four used interaction with peers as their major educational resource for dealing with with these clinical issues. The fifth surgeon used videos from YouTube.

2.8.4 Changes in practice within the past year

All surgeons had made a change in their clinical practice within the last year based on the perception that existing treatment was unsatisfactory. Three surgeons used discussions with colleagues as the educational resource to implement the change. Two attended meetings where they learned about new technology through workshops. In addition one surgeon used an Internet download of a treatment protocol.

2.8.5 Top educational experience

The five surgeons said that their best ever educational experience had been interacting with senior surgeons or peers. These interactions happened during all the stages of their surgical careers, but were most common at the start of independent practice. Interactions usually involved working with a surgeon to solve a problem together.

2.8.6 Printed material use

While all surgeons used books, four used them very extensively. Standard textbooks were the only books in the age of the Internet. Only one surgeon said that books were less important now.

Using journals was very rare. Only one surgeon read journals and only, if he could find an article directly relating to the clinical issue he was trying to address.

2.8.7 Internet use for education

The Internet was used by all of the surgeons to find information about clinical problems and new technology. Accessing new technology was the most interesting feature of the Internet for four of the interviewees. All five used Google as their principal search engine and all were satisfied with its performance. In addition, three used websites of medical device companies containing technical guides. These were felt to be extremely useful.

Two of the surgeons said that they wished to have access to a site that preselected the information they could access. Three of the five would like to talk with other surgeons through the Internet, but all three specified that the discussion must only be with experts. Viewing videos was very popular, as was the ability to look at "live" surgery.

2.8.8 Importance of courses, meetings and symposia

All five surgeons attended their society's annual meeting, an important event for them. All agreed that the interaction they enjoyed with their peers was the most important reason for attending and three of the five felt that social gatherings involving the families were also very important.

All five surgeons attended daily meetings in their hospitals to review the work carried out during that day and all felt that these were very good experiences. None of these meetings were interdisciplinary. In addition, three of the four surgeons attended monthly or bimonthly meetings organized by local societies. These surgeons were very keen to hear speakers from outside.

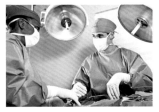

Solving problems together

The five surgeons from Bangladesh said that their best ever educational experience had been interacting with senior surgeons or peers. This was most common at the start of independent practice.

2.8.9   Ease of informal discussions within units

Four of the surgeons felt that informal discussions were easy to arrange within the hospital. The fifth, more senior surgeon, found this difficult to do because he had no colleague of his seniority with whom he could discuss cases.

2.8.10   Importance of product related education

Company representatives regularly visited all of the surgeons. Four surgeons felt that these meetings were extremely useful, particularly with regard to understanding new technology. Workshops were very highly thought of. Only one surgeon felt that these visits were useless.

2.8.11   Existing education facilities and barriers

One of the five surgeons attended a faculty development course, teaching how to create presentation slides.

The hospitals of all the surgeons had libraries, but everyone agreed that these libraries were virtually useless. Three surgeons complained that the hospital Internet was too slow.

Barriers to accessing education were reported by all interviewees. All commented that clinical commitments restricted their ability to attend educational events. Three surgeons felt a lack of finances limited their education.

2.8.12   Suggestions for improving community hospital surgeon education

All the surgeons were convinced that their employing authority could help. Two felt that the hospitals needed to recognize that education was a critical feature for delivering good medical care and that change was essential. Clinical workloads were generally too time consuming for teaching and learning to take place. Three of the surgeons added that good Internet access would be very useful.

2.9   Philippines

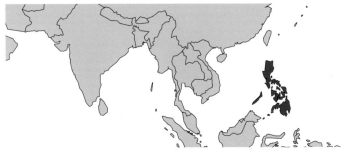

Number of surgeons interviewed

In the Philippines, 6 surgeons with experience ranging from 1 to 25 years past specialist accreditation were interviewed. They came from 4 different hospitals primarily dealing with trauma that also had active orthopedic departments. One of the hospitals was private; 2 were run by the government and 1 by the military. The hospitals served populations of over 500,000 people, except the military hospital. None of the hospitals was a major trauma unit and only the military hospital had surgeons in training.

2.9.1   Why surgeons look for education

All six surgeons agreed that they looked for education to adress clinical problems. Five of the surgeons said that new technology was not an important driver for education, but all were interested in it.

2.9.2   Importance of CPD accreditation

None of the surgeons felt that collecting CPD points was a reason to look for education or enroll in an educational program. Three commented that CPD was completely unimportant to them. One even stated that he did not need to have CPD, but the remaining two surgeons collected CPD points. One surgeon used to collect points but had now given up. Another said one could acquire enough CPD points by merely by attending the annual meeting of the Philippine Orthopaedic Association.

2.9.3   Most recent search for CPD

All interviewees described patients with acute trauma as the most recent reason why they looked for educational help. Five surgeons stated they resolved the clinical problem by talking to peers, the sixth referred to books and used the Internet. One surgeon used books as ancillary help, another searched the Internet.

2.9.4   Changes in practice within the past year

All surgeons incorporated change in at least one aspect of practice. Four surgeons had made the same change in adopting the technique of "Locked Intramedullary Nailing."

Five of the six surgeons had implemented the change after discussions with colleagues. Three of these discussions had taken place at the annual meeting. One occurred during an online alumni network session. One surgeon commented that he was self-taught and the remaining surgeon said that a company representative and technical guides had helped him make the change.

2.9.5   Top educational experience

Three respondents felt that their best ever educational experience was interacting with colleagues. One felt that attending an AO course was his best educational experience and two reported that they were essentially self-taught with the help of books.

2.9.6   Printed material use

The old "standard textbooks" were extensively used by all surgeons.They said reading textbooks helps them to keep up-to-date and get a good over view of specific clinical problems.

Only one of the surgeons used journals on a regular basis, and he needed them only if he could not find the answer in a book. Four surgeons said it was difficult for them to access journals and gave this as the main reason they did not use them more as references.

2.9.7   Internet use for education

While the Internet was used by all six surgeons to access information, their use varied considerably. Finding solutions to clinical problems was the main reason for accessing the Internet, with the exception of one surgeon who

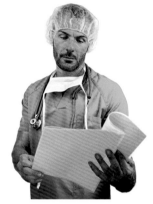

Changes in practice
One surgeon from the Phillipines commented that he was self-taught and one surgeon said that a company representative and the technical guides produced by a commercial company had helped him make the changes.

liked to surf the Internet to see what was new. In terms of search engines, two surgeons used Google, one used Medscape, one used the commercial site by an implant manufacturer. Two surgeons did not use a search engine.

The AO Surgery Reference was used by two surgeons. One surgeon used Pub Med. One surgeon used a commercial website and two surgeons did not mention any websites that were important to them.

When asked what they would like to see in an ideal Internet information source, two of the surgeons were unable to answer the question. The four that did provide answers wanted to be able to read journal articles online and also have access to books. There was a common wish to access a website where minimum navigation was needed to find the requested information. Videos, tips and tricks about the practicalities of surgery were often stated demands for web content.

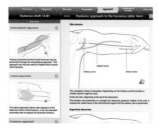

AO Surgery Reference

The AO Surgery Reference was used by two Phillipine surgeons. One surgeon used PubMed. One surgeon used a commercial site and two surgeons had no specific sites that were important to them.

2.9.8   Importance of courses, meetings and symposia

All six surgeons attended national, regional and local meetings. They found the opportunity to talk to colleagues very important and liked the workshops better than the lectures. They saw such meetings as a chance to meet people they did not encounter in their hospital, but only one of the surgeons felt social aspects were important. Attending the annual meeting seems to be a very important educational resource in the Philippines.

There was huge variability in regard to the number and significance of hospital meetings. While five surgeons held meetings in their hospital, the hospital with junior doctors in training had more frequent meetings, and these were felt to be more important from an educational point of view.

2.9.9   Ease of informal discussions within units

Five surgeons reported having major difficulties in holding informal hospital discussions. The most problematic issue was finding the time for chats. Two of the surgeons stated they had difficulty finding a peer in their hospital to have meaningful discussions with.

2.9.10   Importance of product related education

All six surgeons reported regular contact with pharmaceutical and medical device companies, yet none felt that bias was an issue. Five felt that these contacts were important to allow access to new technology. They especially valued the workshops. Four surgeons mentioned that medical educational events would not be possible in the Philippines without financial support from commercial companies.

2.9.11   Existing education facilities and barriers

Four of the surgeons had no educational resources available in the hospital. One hospital had a poor library. Only the large government hospital had a good library and Internet access.

Of the four surgeons who had difficulties attending educational events, financial constraints were a critical factor for three, all of whom said they needed commercial sponsorship otherwise they could not attend an event. The fourth surgeon said that his major constraint was time and he wished educational events were scheduled more on weekends.

2.9.12   Suggestions for improving community hospital surgeon education

Two-thirds of the surgeons wished their hospital would do more to help them. Having experts visit their hospitals was suggested by two people, one wanted protected time to study, and one suggested that the hospital should pay for his education.

Two surgeons saw the solution in the Internet. Both wanted some form of interaction and the ability to contact colleagues and experts to discuss complex cases. They were convinced that this service should be free. Three of the surgeons wished to have heavily subsidized courses, which would be short and focused on workshops. The sixth surgeon wanted short-term fellowships with acknowledged experts.

2.10   Thailand

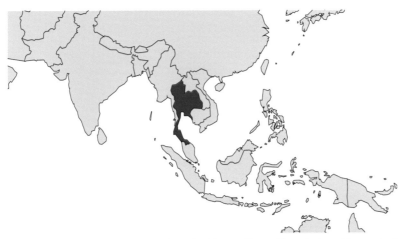

Number of surgeons interviewed

The 4 Thai surgeons interviewed worked in small rural hospitals, with surgical experience ranging from 2 to 17 years post specialist training. The hospitals served populations between 100,000 and 150,000. None of them was a trauma center, however, all took trauma cases. The largest hospital had 6 specialists and one interviewee worked in a solo practice.

2.10.1   Why surgeons look for education

All four surgeons mentioned clinical problems as the reasons they searched for additional education, but they were not particularly interested in new technology. Later in the interviews two of them them came forward with suggestions about learning new technology more rapidly. Although they all worked in small governmental hospitals none had problems getting orthopedic implants if they were clinically indicated.

2.10.2   Importance of CPD accreditation

Collecting CPD points was not important to any of the four surgeons and it was not given as primary motivation for attending an educational event. Two said they did not know which CPD regulations applied to them, but thought that others might know. One surgeon felt that CPD was not important for him; another knew what needed to be done, but said that attending a single meeting a year was sufficient to give him adequate CPD credits.

2.10.3   Most recent search for CPD

All four surgeons identified acute fracture problems as the main reason why they looked for education. Three of the surgeons dealt with the clinical problem by discussing it first with a colleague. One phoned his own chief, one discussed it with a senior person in the hospital and one went to watch a surgeon friend operate in a different hospital. The fourth surgeon accessed information via a company representative who was then present in the operating theatre when the case was dealt with.

2.10.4   Changes in practice within the past year

Last year all four surgeons made at least one change in surgical technique related to orthopedic technology. The surgeons initiated change following discussions with other surgeons. One went to visit a colleague in a different hospital; two contacted surgeon friends in their old teaching institute, and the fourth discussed it with peers while attending a conference.

2.10.5   Top educational experience

Professional interactions were the key to the best educational experiences. All four surgeons liked talking things over with a colleague or experts. However, they were all the opinion that any fruitful discussion must be with somebody that they knew and respected.

2.10.6   Printed material use

Books were important to all the surgeons and two of the four used books, in preference to the Internet, as their first source of information. Standard orthopedic textbooks were used. It was commented that these are very expensive and were often donated by commercial companies.

Three surgeons accessed the "Journal of Bone & Joint Surgery" online. Two of the three read selected articles, but the third surgeon read it cover to cover. One surgeon did not access journals at all.

2.10.7   Internet use for education

The Internet was a good source of information for all interviewees. One surgeon commented that it is the first place to go when he has a clinical problem, but two only used the Internet if they could not find the relevant information in their books.

The preferred search engine for all was Google. Two surgeons used the AO Surgery Reference as their preferred academic website. The third used MD Consult and the fourth went to the website of the Royal College of Surgeons of Thailand.

Three surgeons said that they wanted to watch clinical videos on the Internet. Two would like to have online access to experts either watching live surgery or participating in video conferences. Half of the respondents mentioned issues related to Internet speed. They also wanted the capacity to download full articles.

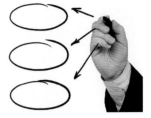

CPD accreditation

Collecting CPD credits was not important to any of the four surgeons from Thailand and it was not a reason for attending an educational event.

2.10.8   Importance of courses, meetings and symposia

Three of the four surgeons attended annual meetings. They saw these events as an opportunity to engage with other doctors and meet colleagues. All three felt that workshops were by far the best aspect of these conferences, apart from professional interaction with peers. None of these surgeons felt that the social aspects of the meeting were important. The fourth surgeon did not find time to get away from his practice to attend any meetings.

2.10.9   Ease of informal discussions within units

Of course, the surgeon in solo practice did not have partners to talk with, but the other three said they had no problems discussing cases with colleagues. However, all of the surgeons commented that they frequently encountered a situation where their colleagues did not have sufficient experience to provide answers. In those cases outside help was needed.

2.10.10   Importance of product related education

All four surgeons reported they had good relationships with commercial companies. They each felt that the representatives from medical device manufacturers helped them access new technology. One went so far as to say that they were by far the best resource available in terms of education. Commercial bias was not an issue. All four surgeons were aware of the potential problem but felt that they did not let commercial bias influence their clinical decision making.

2.10.11   Existing education facilities and barriers

None of the surgeons had received training to be a better teacher or any form of faculty training.

Despite the fact that three of the four hospitals had educational facilities, they were described as a poor, especially the library and the slow Internet. One surgeon said that the meetings held in his hospital were very useful. The fourth surgeon was not aware of any educational resource within his hospital.

While half of interviewees did not have difficulty getting a leave of absence to attend educational courses, the other half did.

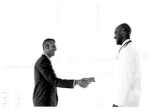

Technology transfer

Close connections with commercial representatives were reported by all four Thai surgeons. They each felt that implant manufacturer representatives were an extremely good resource to allow them access to new technology.

2.10.12   Suggestions for improving community hospital surgeon education

All four surgeons expressed a desire to have more time for education when asked what their hospital could do for them.

Each surgeon wanted more online information about new techniques, new surgical approaches and surgical videos. Two surgeons raised the issue of surgeon-to-surgeon interaction on the web. There was an expressed interest in discussing and sharing cases with other surgeons online.

Interview questions

1. How many years have you been practicing orthopedic surgery as an independent practitioner?

2. What causes you to look for educational opportunities?

   a. Clinical problem (specific)
   b. New Technology (specific)
   c. CPD
   d. Other

3. What last caused you to look for education and how would you describe your recent learning experiences?

4. What sort of teaching characterizes your recent learning experiences?

5. What has been your best educational experience since starting your current job?

6. Have you changed any aspect of your practice in the last year? If so, what was the change and why did you make it?

7. How did you access information / education to allow you to make the change?

8. Do you ever use books in your practice? If so, what causes you to look at a book and how do you access the material?

9. How important are books to your clinical practice?

10. Do you ever use journals in your practice? If so, what causes you to look at a journal and how do you access the material?

11. How important are journals to your practice?

12. Do you use the Internet in your practice? If so, what causes you to access the Internet?

13. How do you access the Internet? Do you use a search engine, and if so which one?

14. Are there any professional websites that you use on a regular basis?

15. How important is the Internet to your practice?

16. What would you really like to have in terms of online learning resources?

17. Do you ever attend formal educational events? If so, what will cause you to do so?

18. How important are formal educational events to your practice?

19. Do you ever attend meetings within the hospital that contribute to your education? If so, what is the purpose of these meetings and how are they organized?

20. Are any of these meetings interdisciplinary? Was the information / education received free from bias? Does this matter to you?

21. Do you have opportunities for discussions with peers or seniors? If so, how are these organized? Could this be made more optimal for you?

22. Do you ever receive education from pharmaceutical or implant manufacturer representatives? If so, why does this happen?

23. Did you find the education you received from commercial sources to be useful in your clinical practice? Did you feel that the information/education given was free from commercial bias? Is freedom from bias important to you?

24. Have you ever received any training to become a more effective teacher and, if so, what was it? Was it helpful in your work? Did you feel it contributed to improved patient care?

25. What resources are you aware exist for education at your hospital?

26. Have you ever encountered any barriers prevented you attending or taking full advantage of available educational resources? If so, what were they and were you able to overcome them?

27. Have you ever encountered any barriers prevented you from putting into practice what you learned at an educational event / meeting? If so, were you able to overcome them?

28. If your employing authority could do one thing that would improve your education to improve the care you give to patients, what would that be?

29. What could anyone do to help you with your education towards improving patient care?

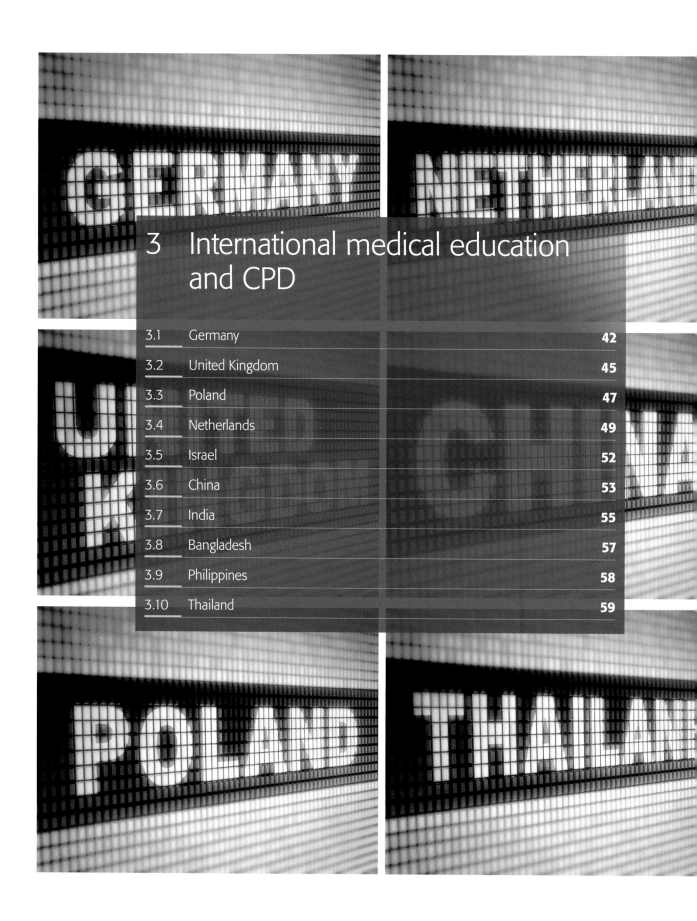

3 International medical education and CPD

3
International medical education and CPD regulation surveys

Surgeon training from medical school through to specialty certification was examined for each of the ten countries involved in the study. To place the educational needs of interviewees into context, the continuing professional development (CPD) regulatory environment was also investigated.

The idea that health professionals have a duty to keep themselves up-to-date and practice medicine to the current acceptable standard is now well established throughout the world. Systems designed to mandate this learning have developed over the past 40 years and continue to evolve.

Initial measures focused on health professionals collecting points for attending approved educational events, carrying out private study or taking part in meetings that were thought to contribute to their learning. The advantages of these systems were that they produced a definable end product that could be verified, for example, Doctor X has devoted 50 hours of his or her time to education in the past year.

These regulatory systems created a huge industry, especially in the United States, whose job it was to ensure educational events met certain standards and could be approved as being suitable for health professional education. The weakness of these systems was that they could only ensure that a given health professional had attended an event. They could not show that an individual had actually learned anything or, more importantly, that attendance had translated into improvements in the health professional's practice that benefited patients.

This study of the educational needs and preferences of surgeons working in community hospitals required understanding how each unique regulatory environment affected surgeons.

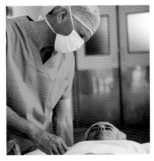

CPD patient benefit?

The weakness of these (regulatory) systems was that they could only ensure that a given health professional had attended an event. They could not show that an individual had actually learned anything.

Information regarding continued professional development (CPD) regulations was obtained from several sources.

- **Internet searches**

  The UK, Germany, Netherlands, India and the Philippines all have national bodies whose websites provided information responsible on regulation of doctors. PubMed searches provided detailed information on the regulatory systems in Israel. Google provided access to information and comment from newspapers in Bangladesh, India and Thailand.

- **Personal questioning of the interviewees**

  All surgeons who were interviewed were asked about the CPD regulations that applied to them. Although most were ignorant of the regulations, several surgeons were able to supply detailed information. This was particularly helpful in Poland and China.

- **Telephone calls**

  The General Medical Council and Royal College of Surgeons of England were contacted by phone because a system of re-accreditation of surgeons is being introduced in the UK that does not involve "point counting". Conversations with these two bodies provided a better understanding of the new regulations.

In addition to the information obtained on CPD regulations, all the surgeons interviewed were asked more general questions about their training and how the medical profession was regarded within their community. These questions were introduced when the pilot study data from the UK and India indicated that social and cultural elements appeared to influence the success of educational programs.

3.1   The medical system in Germany

Medical school length of time	Additional time needed to obtain orthopedic/ trauma certification and independent practice
6 years	6 years plus exam plus license to practice (granted by individual state governments)

[25,26,27,28]

Medical school in Germany takes six years and entry is very competitive. Before medical school begins, it is essential that candidates do an elective on the wards in a nursing assistant's role. Exit examinations are performed in highschool, and only the very best get through. In addition, many medical schools themselves administer a psychological test. All medical schools are government-run and there are no private universities with medical schools. The number of students who wish to enter medical schools is consistently high. Doctors have a very elevated social status.

The first two years of medical school consists of basic science, physics, chemistry, etc. that culminates in an examination. The following three years are spent in hospital doing clinical medicine. The sixth year consists of three periods several months long, one period in internal medicine, one in surgery and one in an elective. All teaching hospitals are linked to universities.

Orthopedics and trauma are now combined in Germany. Previously, trauma was under the realm of general surgery. All training includes general surgery as a stepping stone, then students can pursue internal specialization to include both trauma and orthopedics. These are extremely popular and entry is highly competitive. After six years there is an examination, which leads to a specialist certification valid throughout the European Union.

With this certificate surgeons have a choice: Some stay in hospital as chief resident (German: Oberarzt). The Head of the Department determines the protocols of the unit, but the chief resident is quasi-independent. They can treat patients on their own, but have to justify their decisions and outcomes at daily meetings. Salary levels are vary. The basic salary is between €60,000 and €80,000 a year. In addition, there is some money for being on-call. The main source of extra compensation comes from the chief resident's private earnings. This varies from hospital to hospital. Some chief residents go on to take the equivalent of PhDs and become Professors and Heads of Department, but a significant number of them stay within the medical system and remain perpetual chief residents. As time goes by, there is a tendency for these doctors to become frustrated and some more senior surgeons feel that they only tend to work when they absolutely have to.

A second option for surgeons who complete their specialist certification is to go directly into private practice. To do this, they need to have a license to practice as a specialist; this is determined by the local state government organization. This license allows surgeons to see both government and private patients. The awarding of a certificate depends not only on the competence of the surgeon, but also on the number of doctors who are practicing in the area. As some areas are more popular than others, it can be difficult to get a license there. For example, it is more difficult to get a license in Southern Germany than it is in parts of the former East Germany.

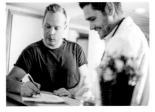

Going into private practice
One option for German surgeons who complete their specialist certification is to go directly into private practice. To do this, they need to have license to practice as a specialist.

There is also the possibility to work in a rehabilitation service. This work consists mainly of checking the work of other doctors and does not require a specialist certification.

3.1.1   CPD regulation in Germany

CPD requirements * not applicable to private system	Accreditation organizations	Non-compliance consequences
50 points per year; 250 every 5 years; 150 within specialty (points related to hours of teaching)	- German Medical Association - 17 regional "Medical Chambers"	- Financial sanctions (fee reduction) - Withdrawal of license after two years

In 2004, a major reform of quality management and CPD took place in Germany through the Social Health Insurance (SHI) Modernization Act (Gesetz zur Modernisierung der gesetzlichen Krankenversicherung). Amongst other things, this Act made CPD compulsory for all physicians, apart from those who are purely private (ie, not funded by SHI). While CPD is mandatory, the German CPD system is a complex one, not least because various bodies are involved in the management, implementation and quality assurance of CPD. Due to the system of sixteen states (Länder) in Germany there are actually seventeen (two in one of the largest states) primary organizations involved in overseeing CPD, with some 500 professional CPD providers. Each state in Germany is able to issue individual standards on CPD, although those are fairly homogenous across Germany.

The German parliament (specifically the Ministry of Health) sets the legal framework for health care provision in Germany. Its Joint Committee issues standardized and binding directives in order to translate the legal framework into practice. It delegates responsibility for CPD to the German Medical Association.

The Bundesärztekammer (the German Medical Association) is the federal medical association with overall responsibility for issuing core guidance on the CPD system. It has issued a model regulatory framework to all seventeen regional Medical Chambers of Physicians (Ärztekammer), which authorize their own CPD programs, approve CPD courses or seminars in their region, and decide how many credit points each CPD activity merits.

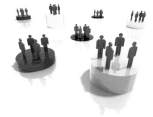

Various groups involved

While CPD is mandatory, the German CPD system is a complex one, not least because there are various bodies which are involved in the management, implementation and quality assurance of CPD.

CPD accreditation does not exist in the private system, although there are plans to see if it can be introduced. For doctors who treat government patients there are strict CPD guidelines, mainly acquiring points to prove that the doctors are up-to-date with their education. The points are related to the hours of teaching received and do not reflect quality or the effectiveness of the teaching. Doctors are often free to choose the activities they participate in, although there are exceptions. Sherry Merkur et al. write in their article "Physician revalidation in Europe" (Cinical Medicine 2008) that "specialists working in hospital have to show that 70% of their vocational training has been on topics concerning their specialty."

A recent presentation by the director of the Regional Chamber Hessen (Landesärztekammer) essentially confirms this, stating that 150 CPD credits must be gained in topics specific to the doctors' specialty, with the other 100 CPD credits from topics of their choice. GPs and specialists working in ambulatory care do not have any restrictions placed on the CPD topics they can cover.

Physician membership in their regional association is mandatory to qualify for reimbursement through the statutory health insurance system. Ambulatory care doctors must report their CPD points to their regional association in order to maintain their license to work within the social health insurance system. This suggests that those who fail to do so will have their license revoked. According to one source, if doctors are non-compliant with the CPD requirements, doctors face "strict financial sanctions (fee reductions) and withdrawal of [their] license after two years."

Almost every Regional Chamber has introduced an online CPD system to help doctors record their CPD activity. Each doctor is given their own 15-digit "uniform CPD number" (einheitliche Fortbildungsnummer, EFN), an identification card and a set of personal barcode stickers. When doctors apply for a CPD activity, they place one of their barcode stickers on the application, which is then scanned at the event. The CPD points are immediately added to the physician's online account, meaning they do not need to fill in any paperwork themselves. This system has been in place since October 2005, and according to one source "is working out quite well."

An article by Schlette and Klemperer (2009) [29] suggests that there are various problems with CPD in Germany. Apparently, "CME and quality management systems were introduced by the government against the will of the professional bodies, yet implementation and oversight fall under the latter's remit." Moreover, CPD and quality management requirements are not aimed at identifying poor or harmful practitioners. More modern, internationally recognized models of CPD still have not entered the medical community's language beyond lip-service.

In summary, Germany's complex CPD system consists of the following: CPD is compulsory for the vast majority of doctors in Germany. The main body which issues guidance on CPD is the German Medical Association.

There are 16 states in Germany, each of which has a Chamber with its own ability to set standards on mandatory CPD. However, the German Medical Association issues national guidelines in an attempt to standardize CPD. Generally, CPD is run on a five-year cycle.

Specialists are required to undertake the majority of their CPD in specialty-specific subjects. Doctors must gain 50 CPD points per year. A system of accrediting CPD events exists, but the robustness of this system has been questioned. Germany is the only country that has introduced a barcode system for doctors, through which CPD providers can automatically scan doctors' attendance onto a database.

3.2   The medical system in the United Kingdom

Medical school length of time	Additional time needed to obtain orthopedic/ trauma certification and independent practice
5–6 years plus 2 year Foundation program	6 years plus exam

[30]

Entry into UK medical school is highly competitive. Candidates are required to have high academic qualifications and many schools require candidates complete exams designed to test problem-solving skills.

Medical school lasts 5–6 years and is followed by a two year "Foundation Programme" where the doctor is closely supervised and rotated through a number of specialties. Successful completion of this two-year program leads to the award of a Foundation Achievement of Competence Document (FACD).

Once a FACD has been obtained doctors may apply for entry into orthopedic specialist training, which is highly competitive. The training takes six years and ends with an examination: FRCS (ORTH).

3.2.1   CPD regulation in the UK

CPD requirements	Accreditation organizations	Non-compliance consequences
250 credits every 5 year cycle; 50 credits per year (1 credit per hour)	- Academy of Medical Royal Colleges - Specialist colleges	Revalidation may be denied

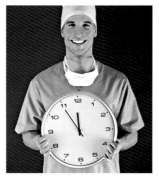

Measured in hours
In the new UK system CPD is measured in hours, with appropriate developmental activity measured hour for hour. Surgeons are responsible for recording the CPD activity.

The new UK system of CPD is intimately connected to the concept of revalidation/recertification and is in an early stage of evolution. Here, CPD is measured in hours, with appropriate developmental activity measured hour for hour. Surgeons are responsible for recording the CPD activity and the hours that are attributed to it and expected to accrue at least 50 hours per year and a minimum of 250 hours every five years of their revalidation cycle. There is some flexibility from year to year at the discretion of appraisers.

Three categories of activities and environments have been designated to help achieve balance throughout a surgeon's Personal Development Plan (PDP): clinical. academic and professional activities in an internal, external and peronal environment. There are no limits on the number of hours that can be claimed for the same type of activity. However, to encourage a balanced program, normally no more than 20 of the minimum 50 hours per year should come from a single type of activity.

It is the responsibility of individual doctors to engage in good quality, balanced CPD activities that complement both their practice and learning needs. Self-accreditation is encouraged and allowed. Uniquely, the UK CPD system has made room for flexibility in what is defined as learning. In situations where doctors have self-accredited an activity, evidence of the education activity is required and may consist of documented reflection.

Surgeons can track their CPD activities online using the Surgeon's Portfolio tool that allows for the upload of certificates and other proof of learning, including a section for reflection on all activities using standard questions. Organizations are piloting methods of estimating the educational value of CPD activities that would, in the future, help relate credits to the quality of learning achieved.

Under the new scheme, all doctors who have a license to practice will be required to provide documentation that they are participating in CPD in order to keep up-to-date and fit to practice. Documentation that one has participated in and learned from CPD events with set standards will be a requirement for revalidation.

Surgeons are free to participate in the CPD systems of any of the three UK surgical colleges. A charge is levied for non-members.

3.3   The medical system in Poland

Medical school length of time	Additional time needed to obtain orthopedic/ trauma certification and independent practice
6 years plus 1 year internship	5 year residency (will not lead to independent practice if doctor remains in Poland) plus exam

[31,32,33]

In Poland, medicine is not highly regarded as a good career choice as there is an over-production of doctors. When Poland was part of the Warsaw Pact the country was responsible for the training of all armed forces doctors. The military medical school has survived. The surgeons interviewed feel that there is one medical school too many in Poland.

Studying medicine lasts for six years and entry to medical school is competitive. Following graduation, all doctors must complete one year compulsory training in a hospital. Six months is spent in internal medicine, two months in obstetrics and gynecology, two months in pediatrics, and two months in surgery, including both orthopedics and traumatology.

Following this one year of compulsory training, doctors enter a residency program lasting five years, three and a half years of which is in orthopedics and traumatology. The rest of the time is reserved for other surgical subjects, including general surgery, neurosurgery, urology, cardiothoracic surgery, ICU and rehabilitation. Although entry into this program is competitive, all applicants get a place within two years providing they are prepared to travel some distance to other hospitals.

Residency training is organized according to the county you come from. In theory, it is possible to enter a residency program outside your home area but in practice this rarely happens. At the start of residency, there are numerous courses organized both locally and nationally. They are lecture dominated and have not significantly changed in the last decade. They are not highly regarded.

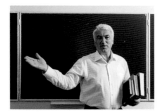

At the end of residency, there is an examination that consists of multiple choice questions (MCQ) and a clinical oral examination. In theory, there is also a practical examination where surgeons are observed during an operation but in practice this does not happen and this part of the exam is carried out largely by telephone calls between superiors.

Lectures dominate

In Poland, at the start of residency, there are numerous courses organized both locally and nationally. The characteristics of these courses are that they are lecture dominated and have not significantly changed in the last decade.

After residency large numbers of doctors do not get jobs and there has been a huge migration of doctors, particularly to other countries within the European Union. The education system for residents has not evolved in any significant way in the last few years.

If doctors stay in Poland, they usually are employed in an assistant's post and do not go into independent practice.

3.3.1   CPD regulation in Poland

CPD requirements	Accreditation organizations	Non-compliance consequences
200 points every 2 years (200 hours)	Supreme Medical Council (NIL)	- Not enforced - May impact recruitment (Doctors have boycotted the system for the past 6 years)

In theory, Poland has very strict CPD regulations. Doctors must collect 200 points within a two year period by attending educational events, writing articles, attending departmental meetings, etc., and most can collect sufficient points. They then are required to present their portfolio of learning to the doctor's chapter. One point is awarded for each hour of study.

Doctors registered with the medical chambers are obliged by law—Law on Doctor Professions (Ustawa o zawodzie lekarza) and Ministry of Health Decree from 2004—to revalidate their license (in the Polish context it is called the recertification process). However, as stated by interviewees, there are no direct sanctions if doctors do not observe this law. There are some control procedures and medical chambers may advise a doctor to retrain (eg, in cases where a doctor has not practiced medicine for longer than five years), but in practice, once a medical license has been granted it cannot be revoked (except under specific circumstances).

The certification/accreditation of organizations providing continuous professional training/postgraduate training in medicine is the responsibility of the Supreme Medical Council (Naczelna Izba Lekarska (NIL)). The NIL (through its Committee for Medical Education) also keeps a register of all accredited education providers

Although, as stated, there are no direct sanctions imposed on doctors who do not participate in further training, the NIL is often consulted during the recruitment of senior medical practitioners. On these occasions, lack of evidence of a doctor's recertification acts to his or her disadvantage and the NIL may advise hospitals and other medical providers not to appoint particular candidates.

The surgeons who were interviewed feel that the system does not work because the doctors have boycotted it for the past six years, citing problems with the system's administration. Administrative clerks did not recognize what constituted relevant training. There was also the issue that many doctors could not afford to attend the three to four competency courses a year to aquire the necessary 200 points. In private institutions, the hospital director takes care of doctor training.

3.4   The medical system in the Netherlands

Medical school length of time	Additional time needed to obtain orthopedic/ trauma certification and independent practice
6 years	variable

[34,35,36]

Entry into medical school is highly competitive and the majority of medical students are now women [37]. Undergraduate medical training takes six years in the Netherlands and ends with a final licensing examination, which bestows the university degree of Medical Doctor, the formal qualification to practice medicine.

Registration as a medical doctor in accordance with the Individual Health Care Professions Act is a prerequisite for a specialist training post. Dutch specialist training is characterized by the presence of an elaborately regulated and closely monitored training system, where the focus is on practical training; there is an absence of a specialist exam. Regulations for specialist training mainly concern requirements for the specialists in charge of training at teaching hospitals/institutions and concern the duration, content and conditions of the training. They are proposed by the organizations of the various medical specialties to ensure content validity and public support.

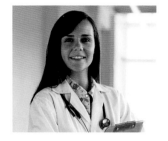

More female students
In the Netherlands entry into medical school is highly competitive and the majority of medical students are now women. Undergraduate medical training takes six years.

All surgical trainees are required to complete a basic period of training during which they rotate through all the major surgical specialties. One of these rotations is in orthopedics and trauma, and part of that rotation includes attendance at an AO Principles course. This means that a gynecologist who will never practice orthopedics has to attend an AO course as part of their training.

The basic assumption of the system is that specialist training can only be provided by recognized specialists in approved training hospitals. Only doctors working in a hospital/institution, recognized as a training hospital, are eligible for recognition as head of training in that specialty.

To be recognized as head of training, the specialist must have been registered in his or her specialty for at least five years and have adequate practical experience. They also must provide evidence of organizational skills and prove their research meets current standards of medical ethics.

A doctor who plans to enter training in a specialist program has to apply for a training place at a specialist-training department. If accepted by the trainer, he or she is required to notify the Committee for the Registration of Medical Specialists (MSRC) and to submit a training schedule for approval. This schedule must be in accordance with regulations for the specialty concerned. The trainee works as a resident under the supervision of a trainer. Over the course of the training, the resident should gradually assume greater responsibility.

Training consists of a theoretical and a practical part. The relative importance of practice and theory varies from specialty to specialty and is laid down in the teaching rules. At the end of each year of training, the trainer sends an evaluation of the resident to the MSRC. In the case of problems concerning the resident's progress, the MSRC is empowered to rule that the resident must prolong, or even terminate, the training.

Having completed the training, the MSRC may, on receipt of the trainer's final statement, enter the resident in the Dutch register of specialists. The resident must provide the MSRC with detailed information about the training in form of a logbook. As one of the requirements for registration, he or she must publish a paper in a peer-reviewed journal or present a lecture at a peer-reviewed scientific meeting. Once registered, he or she has to practice on a regular basis for 16 hours a week and attend 40 hours of formal continuing medical education each year to be reregistered for another 5 years.

According to the Individual Healthcare Professions Act (BIG Act, wet op de beroepen in de individuele gezondheidszorg) only practitioners who comply with the training and education requirements for their profession may be registered in the BIG register. Registration is conducted through the Ministry of Health, Welfare and Sport, via the BIG register. The Royal Dutch Medical Association (KNMG) is not involved in the initial registration and licensing of physicians.

While there is no national licensing exam, there are certain conditions doctors must meet before being included in the BIG register, among them:

• They must hold a valid diploma.

• They must be permitted to practice the profession without restrictions.

• They must pay the appropriate registration fee.

• They must not have been placed under supervision due to a psychological disorder.

There are two types of medical licenses issued in the Netherlands: a provisional license, whereby professionals are permitted to work under supervision for a two year period before obtaining full registration, and full registration, which allows independent practice for an indefinite period, subject to re-accreditation.

3.4.1   CPD regulation in the Netherlands

CPD requirements	Accreditation organizations	Non-compliance consequences
40 hours per year plus minimum work quotas (plus 2 hours peer review each year for general practitioners)	- Royal Dutch Medical Association (KNMG) - Specialist organizations	Re-registration not granted

The formal CPD authority in the Netherlands is the KNMG (Royal Dutch Medical Association). In 2002, over thirty professional specialist societies, the three Registration Committees (medical specialists, social medicine doctors, GPs and nursing home doctors) came together to create the KNMG. This was "to develop a harmonized system of accreditation of continuing medical education and awarding of credits."

Accreditation of CPD remains the responsibility of the separate professional societies. According to the KNMG, "establishing a central national continuing education authority is not contemplated." However, in order to standardize accreditation of CPD events, a uniform application form and assessment framework has been used by all the professional societies since November 2004.

In 1996, it became a requirement for general practitioners and specialist doctors to re-register every five years. In that year, the requirements for reregistration were a minimum of eight hours a week of medical work, participation in 40 hours accredited CPD per year and participation in one peer review every five years. An online system called GAIA has been developed for doctors to record their CPD activities. The requirements have changed over the past fifteen years. Currently, in order for general practitioners to reregister it is compulsory that they do the following:

Demonstrate that they have undertaken at least 16 hours of general practice work in every week during the previous five years. Since 2009, GPs also had to demonstrate that they have undertaken 50 hours of evening, night or weekend work per year.

They must have taken at least 40 hours of accredited CPD each year for five years.

From January 2009, CPD had to include at least two hours "visitatie" or peer review per year. As of January 1, 2010, peer review was only recognized if a specialist consultant GP with a supervision qualification approved by the College of Specialist GPs, accompanied the peer review.

For specialists to reregister it is compulsory that they complete the following: For medical geriatric, psychiatric and GP specialists: demonstrate that they have worked for at least 16 hours per week in their specialty. If the above is not achieved, doctors must have collected at least 200 hours of accredited CPD in the previous five years.

It would appear from the data collected that participation in the peer review scheme is not yet a requirement for the reregistration of specialists.

Should doctors fail to comply with CPD, there is the possibility to reregister doctors for a shorter period (for example, one year). During this time, the doctors should make up the CPD hours they were missing. Doctors must then attempt to re-register at the end of this period.

The system of "visitatie" (peer review) was established in the Netherlands in the 1990s "as a way of ensuring the quality of patient services and to reconfirm the trust of the public, financiers, and government in the self-regulating mechanism of the profession. "The 27 medical specialty societies in the Netherlands developed and executed the "visitatie" system, which is a doctor-led and doctor-owned peer review system aimed at assessing the

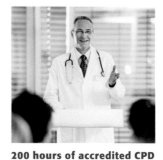

200 hours of accredited CPD
In 1996, it became a requirement for Dutch GP and specialist doctors to re-register every five years. Currently, in order for GPs to re-register it is compulsory that they have undertaken at least 40 hours of accredited CPD each year for five years.

quality of medical practice of hospital-based specialist groups. As stated above, it is currently only compulsory for GPs.

In summary, the Netherland's CPD/re-registration system consists of the following:

- CPD is compulsory for GPs and specialists, but is not for non-specialist doctors. It is directly linked to a system of recertification, which has been referred to as revalidation.

- Doctors must take part in 40 hours of CPD per year, and GPs must take part in at least two hours peer review per year.

- There is little information available on the peer review of CPD. However, it has recently been made compulsory for a trained specialist GP to attend peer review meetings.

- The framework for accreditation has also been standardized on a national level.

3.5   The medical system in Israel

Medical school length of time	Additional time needed to obtain orthopedic/ trauma certification and independent practice
6 years plus 1 year internship	6 years post-registration program plus exam

[38,39]

In Israel, the Ministry of Health is the responsible government body for granting medical licenses (1976 Physician's Ordinance). After completing six years of university medical school, graduates must complete a 12-month internship, for which they receive a medical diploma. They may then apply for a permanent medical license through the Division of Medical Professions at the Ministry of Health. Israel does not have mandatory relicensure or reregistration. Physicians who study in Israel are not required to take a licensing exam.

In addition to six years of medical education, plus an internship year (and exam, where relevant), the law requires each license applicant to be an "upstanding human being" (usually defined as having no criminal record), be an Israeli citizen or permanent resident, and have a basic command of the Hebrew language. Registration with the Israeli Medical Association (IMA) is not mandatory; nevertheless, the majority of publicly employed physicians are members of the IMA.

Acceptance in post-registration programs is highly competitive and involves psychomotoric testing. For orthopedic training candidates have to spend four years on orthopedics/trauma and another two years on different subjects such as intensive care and general surgery. Residents are trained within a single hospital. Entry into orthopedic training is competitive, but variable. Certain large hospitals have high demand and some smaller units do not.

Every hospital within the state system employs residents and every orthopedic department within the state system is responsible for their training. Training is based in the resident's hospital, although there are some weekly postgraduate seminars organized by universities for the whole of Israel. Efforts are made to arrange some common resident meetings every two months in the south of Israel, but this has not happened yet.

Although a formal curriculum and exit exam exists, the vast majority of training is based on the patients that the doctor sees during any working day. Although a single consultant is appointed to to be in overall charge of the residents, every consultant in every hospital working within the Israeli state system is responsible for postgraduate education.

Within the private sector there are a small numbers of hospitals, which do not have residents, and therefore there is no formal educational program.

3.5.1   CPD regulation in Israel

CPD requirements	Accreditation organizations	Non-compliance consequences
Israel does not have a CPD system.		

There is no formal CPD accreditation process in Israel. Consultants are not required to take any time off for formal education during their working day/week. There is no system for evaluating consultants, no appraisal or assessment. Proposals to introduce such a system are missing. It follows that CPD accreditation is unimportant to Israeli consultants.

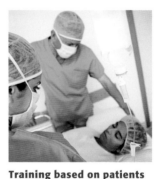

Training based on patients
Although there is a formal curriculum and exit exam for Israeli doctors, the vast majority of training is based on the patients that the doctor sees during any working day.

3.6   The medical system in China

Medical school length of time	Additional time needed to obtain orthopedic/ trauma certification and independent practice
5–7 years	4 year Masters plus PhD program (dissertation)

[40,41]

At the age of 18, pupils must pass an exit exam from secondary school to be admitted to colleges and other places of further education. Entry to medical school depends on the marks achieved. Getting into a good medical school is very competitive and high school exam scores must be extremely high. Despite these hurdles, doctors do not have a particularly high status in China. Doctors who practice internal medicine have low salaries. Orthopedic doctors have higher salaries and entry into orthopedic training is therefore much more competitive than for most other specialties.

Medical school lasts between five and seven years depending on the course studied. Teaching in medical school is primarily done through lectures and practical studies in connection with anatomy. Although questions and answers are common at the end of lectures, there is very little opportunity for discussion, which is not encouraged. There is a lot of book learning and the examinations are based on repeating what has been written in books. The biggest difference between education in the West and China is that discussion does not feature in Chinese education. In internal medicine for example, candidates are expected to memorize 1,200 pages of a book.

Only the final year of medical school is spent in the hospital and medical students do not see a patient until this point. At the end of medical school, they get a certificate of completion. There is no final examination.

Immediately after leaving medical school, doctors can enter a three-year study for a master's degree in orthopedics after taking a competitive entrance examination. Work is a mixture of practical training and research, followed a year as an intern. There is no formal rotation nor a final orthopedic examination, but students are expected to produce a final dissertation.

Having completed the master's course, surgeons either become a lecturer in a big teaching hospital or continue to a PhD. Entrance into the PhD program depends on the results of a difficult exam. If an orthopedic trainee chooses to be a lecturer in a big hospital, he or she will work under supervision and may continue to do for the rest of their career. After the master's examination there is no possibility to enter into independent practice. If a surgeon wishes to get a job as a professor he or she must complete a PhD.

Most doctors practice in government hospitals. There are very few private practices, although this is changing. Current salaries in government hospitals vary. Every doctor has a fixed salary and gets some payment for overtime. Commissions are received from device manufacturers and pharmaceutical firms. This is unofficial but common.

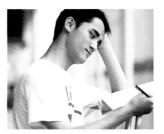

Learning from books

The biggest difference between education in the West and China is that discussion does not feature prominently in Chinese education. There is a lot of book learning and the examinations are based on repeating what has been written in books.

3.6.1 CPD regulation in China

Required hours of CPD	Accreditation organizations	Non-compliance consequences
25 hours per year	Local societies, governmental bodies	Rarely administered outside a few teaching hospitals

Every doctor in China is expected to complete 25 hours of CPD approved education each year. In practice, this is very rarely enforced outside a small number of teaching hospitals. CPD accreditation is left to local societies, as well as to governmental bodies. Most CPD events consist of lectures. Getting access to CPD approved education is not difficult if the surgeon works in a government hospital.

Most Chinese doctors wish to keep themselves up-to-date and feel that the difficulty in accessing medical information and technology from outside China and lack of access to this information is a major obstruction to their personal and professional development. Consequently the biggest and most common wish of all Chinese doctors is to travel outside China to complement their medical education.

3.7   The medical system in India

Medical school length of time	Additional time needed to obtain orthopedic/ trauma certification and independent practice
4.5 years plus 1 year internship	3 years plus exam

[42,43,44,45]

There are not enough doctors for India's growing population. This is one of the reasons why Indian doctors have a very high status. There is also a tradition of respect dating back several hundred years. Doctors were once part of the royal court. They treated their patients for free, and were in return paid by their rulers. Doctors' current salaries make them members of the upper middle class.

Entry into medical school is very competitive. Less than 1% of applicants are accepted. Medical school in India consists of four and a half years of study followed by one year of internship. The pre-clinical course lasts two years, and is divided into topics such as anatomy, physiology, and others. This is followed by clinical training which lasts two and a half years. On any given day, medical students will see up to 100 patients in the outpatient clinic. At the end of medical school, there is a final examination consisting of essays, short notes and clinical examinations. MCQ-type examinations (multiple choice) are only just being introduced.

The one-year internship or Compulsory Rotatory Residential Internship (CRRI) consists of four three-month clinical attachments in medicine, including psychiatry; surgery (with A & E, accident and emergency) and anesthesia. One month of the surgical rotation is devoted to orthopedics and trauma. Obstetrics, gynecology and pediatrics; and community medicine (The 4th clinical attachment), are taught outside the hospital. The hours are very long and there is only a one-day leave per month. At the end of the one year internship, doctors are registered with the Indian Medical Council. This allows them to set up their own practice, as well as do accident and emergency, minor surgery, normal obstetric delivery and emergency Caesarean sections.

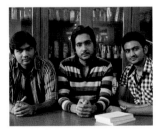

In India entry into medical school is very competitive. Less than 1% of applicants are accepted. Medical school ensists of four and a half years of study followed by one year of internship.

Specializing in any surgical field will allow a doctor to earn more money, orthopedics being a very lucrative specialty. In India, it is still possible to earn a good living from treating trauma. At this point, the doctor has three choices if they wish to pursue a career in orthopedics and traumatology.

1) Take a competitive exam held by the national examination board to gain a place in orthopedics and traumatology training. (For this a primary exam during internship must first be completed) This examination exists for all medical specialties, not just orthopedics and traumatology. Having passed the examination successfully, the doctor may then be sent to work in a remote hospital.

2) The postgraduate orthopedics route. This is a very limited option with only 20 to 25 spaces available in each state. There is an examination, where preference is given to minority groups. The postgraduate medical scheme provides the same sort of training as the one given by the national examination board, but the degree is from a university, not the board.

3) The third possibility is to go overseas for training, which is usually done in the United Kingdom, Canada, United States, New Zealand, and Australia.

Specialized training in orthopedics and traumatology takes three years. Successfully passing the final exam bestows the titel of master of surgery. After completing the course, surgeons have three career possibilities:

A) Surgeons can start their own hospital. This is a popular option if the surgeons parents are doctors. The decision to set up a private hospital depends on finances only.

B) Surgeons can join the government service, working in the city hospitals as an assistant surgeon.

C) Surgeons can join a corporate hospital as a member of staff. These hospitals can give the surgeon a greater degree of autonomy than government service.

3.7.1   CPD regulation in India

CPD requirements	Accreditation organizations	Non-compliance consequences
38 hours every 5 years	Medical Council of India	System not yet implemented

The Medical Council of India has specified that every doctor has to have 38 hours of CPD every five years when working in the government system [46,47,48]. This system, however, is not yet implemented and surgeons and other health professionals do not have to produce documentary evidence of CPD.

Nevertheless, there is a complex system of awarding CPD accreditations for medical events. This system is based on specialist, national and state societies that submit their event programs to the appropriate licensing authority. The surgeons are awarded CPD credit points [49] based on attendance. These points are generally not perceived as important for an individual's educational portfolio or his or her ability to continue practice.

3.8   The medical system in Bangladesh

Medical school length of time	Additional time needed to obtain orthopedic/ trauma certification and independent practice
5 years plus mandatory 1 year internship	4–5 years post medical school in Masters or Fellowship program plus 4–5 years work in public sector

[50]

Medicine is viewed as a very prestigious career in Bangladesh. Entry to medical school is highly competitive and is based on the results of the candidate's Higher School Certificate. Less than 10% of applicants are admitted to either private or government medical school. Entry into government medical schools is more competitive than to private ones as the fees are much lower. Additionally, acquiring patients is more difficult in the private sector. Medical school lasts 5 years and there is a final exam.

All doctors must complete a one year internship after leaving medical school during which the doctor rotates through all the specialties. Training in orthopedics and trauma can be obtained via two routes: a Master's degree at a university or a fellowship program through the College of Physicians. Courses vary in length, but 4-5 years is normal with 2 years being devoted to general surgery.

Having completed specialist training surgeons can work in the public or private sectors. Progress to full independent practice may take a further 5-6 years in the public sector.

3.8.1   CPD regulations in Bangladesh

CPD requirements	Accreditation organizations	Non-compliance consequences
Bangladesh does not currently have a CPD system.		

Although the College of Physicians and the government are keen to introduce a CPD system in Bangladesh, it does not exist yet and there are no plans to implement one in the near future.

Bangladeshi doctors, on the other hand, expressed keen interest in medical education and in developing a national CPD system. In 2012 A Whobab Khan, associate professor at the Bangabandhu Sheikh Mujib Medical University in Dhaka wrote in the Bangladeshi Journal of Medical Education, "We need to improve ourselves to cope with the changing working environment. As an adult learner the effective CPD program and the guideline for us is still wanting for our country. And for that we need to find out the answer of many basic questions like what is the attitude of our doctors for life long learning and how they think to change their practice. How and why they will be motivated to take positive steps to CPD. As there is no definite guideline from the regulatory body or the policy maker authority

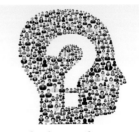

Many basic questions

"And for that we need to find out the answer of many basic questions like what is the attitude of our doctors for life long learning and how they think to change their practice."
Professor MA Wohab Khan, Bangabandhu Sheikh Mujib Medical University, Dhaka, Bangladesh.

in many developing countries like ours; the professional organizations should come forward to formulate the research to provide information for developing a motivation in personal and organizational level and should develop a guideline and implement the CPD program among the members. And the most important is that there should be a combined and collaborative effort to convince, motivate and guide the policy makers and accrediting authority." [51]

3.9   The medical system in the Philippines

Medical school length of time	Additional time needed to obtain orthopedic/ trauma certification and independent practice
4 year BSc plus 4 years plus 1 year senior internship	4 years plus exam

[52]

Doctors are very well regarded in the Philippines. They have a high status and enjoy a great deal of respect. Although they are reasonably well paid, their salaries are not as high as those of politicians and businessmen.

Phillipine medical education is closely based on the United States system. All people entering medical school have completed four years of college and hold a BSc degree. This is followed by four years in either a private or government run medical school. Entry into medical school is controlled by national medical examinations and the passing rate is approximately 50%. Students must pay for their own education and scholarships are extremely rare. Medical school demands four years of study, the fourth year as an intern. In the second year students start seeing patients. There is a senior internship in year five, which consists of working on the wards. This is always closely supervised. Medical training ends with an examination.

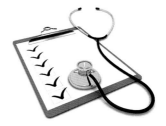

Rigorous examinations
At the end of each year Fillipino orthopedic trainees have an examination and the candidates cannot pass on to the next year of training unless they have passed that exam. There is also an exit examination.

Entry into orthopedic training is extremely competitive. The programs consist of four years of training in orthopedics and orthopedic traumatology. During these four years, trainees rotate through all orthopedic subspecialties. At the end of each year, they have to take an exam and the candidates cannot move on to the next year of training unless they have passed that exam. There is also an exit examination at the end.

Having successfully passed the exit examination, doctors may go to work in a government hospital. If they do that, they go in as a Medical Officer Grade IV. This post does not involve performing operations unsupervised, although the degree of supervision is variable. Staying within the government system allows the doctors to progress through different ranks of Medical Officer and they may eventually enter private practice, which many people choose to do. Surgeons in the major centers often carry out a combination of government and private work. Most government contracts allow practitioners to do a certain amount of private work which pays significantly more than government service. Private practice pays significantly more than government service.

3.9.1 CPD regulation in the Philippines

CPD requirements	Accreditation organizations	Non-compliance consequences
25 hours per year	- Philippine Orthopaedic Association - Royal College - College of Surgeons	* System currently in dispute and not functioning

The Philippine Orthopaedic Association used to be responsible for CPD accreditation. Doctors were expected to get 25 hours per year of approved CPD activities [53]. At present, there is a dispute as to who is going to manage the system as both the Royal College and the College of Surgeons wish to have this role. As a result, the CPD accreditation system in the Philippines has fallen into abeyance and there is, in fact, no current control over CPD regulations for doctors practicing orthopedics within the Philippines.

3.10   The medical system in Thailand

Medical school length of time	Additional time needed to obtain orthopedic/ trauma certification and independent practice
6 years plus 1 year working internship plus 2 year working internship	4 years plus board exam

[54,55]

Doctors enjoy a very high status in Thailand and admission to medical school is highly competitive, making it very difficult to gain entrance. The program lasts six years: a year of basic sciences, then two years of clinical sciences, followed by a three-year clinical course. After medical school, all doctors must complete 2 internships: a one year internship in their teaching institute, plus two years working in a hospital away from the main centers. There, doctors rotate through all the specialties, including general practice.

Entering orthopedic residency is very competitive. Orthopedic trainees are generally based in a single hospital, but may have duties outside to learn other aspects of surgery. The orthopedic residency lasts four years, with a board exam at the end.

Orthopedic trainees may be attached to small peripheral hospitals where they work in independent practice at a very early stage in their career. Trainees working in larger units have much greater supervision.

Salaries are based on civil servant salaries. A surgeon's salary depends on the number of hours worked. The private sector is usually a more lucrative option, but being employed by the government includes extra benefits such as children's education and healthcare.

3.10.1   CPD regulation in Thailand

CPD requirements	Accreditation organizations	Non-compliance consequences
Thailand does not currently have a CPD system		

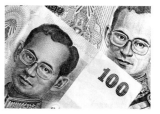

In Thailand a surgeon's salary depends on the number of hours worked. The private sector is usually more lucrative, but being employed by the government includes extra benefits.

In 2008, the World Health Organization held a conference in Chiang Mai [56] to draw up guidelines for a system of CPD regulation that could be applied to countries in South East Asia. These guidelines have not yet been implemented in Thailand, but individual events are accredited by specialist organizations such as the Royal College of Orthopaedic Surgeons of Thailand.

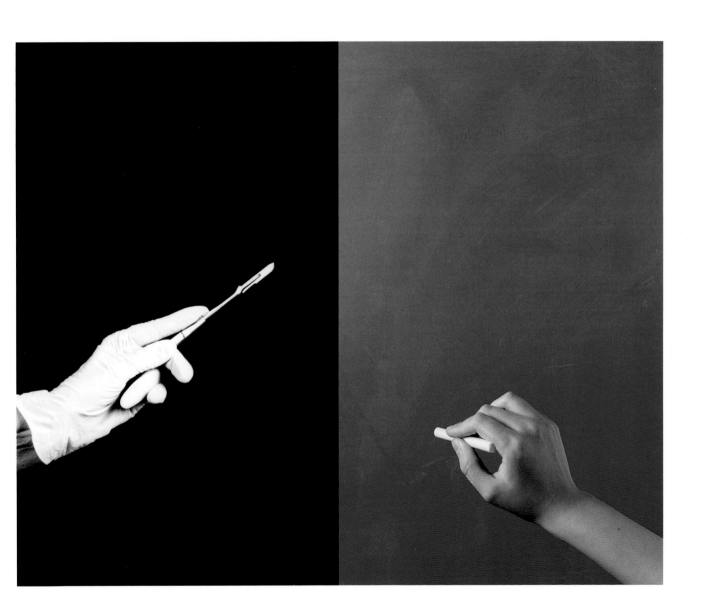

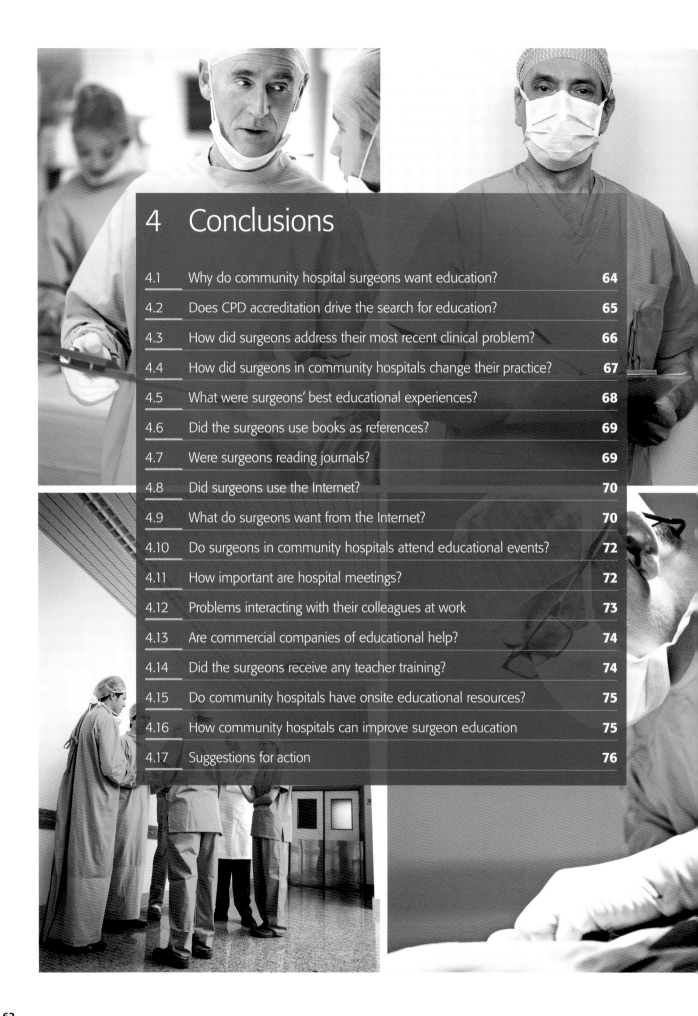

4 Conclusions

4
Conclusions: how surgeons in community hospitals approach learning

Time constraints and financial limitations impede community hospital surgeons' desire to take courses or attend events. The Internet may appear to be a perfect medium for information delivery but those practicing in the developing world encounter serious barriers accessing this technology.

The introduction of new techniques and technologies advances orthopedic and trauma surgery at an ever hastening pace. This inexorable march of progress means that surgeons need to continually evaluate their current practices and update them when needed. Patients, health care providers and insurers expect surgeons to educate themselves throughout their professional lives. Although experience is still a key factor associated with successful practice, patients now expect experience to be combined with training in the latest knowledge and skills.

Medicine has always had centers of excellence, which have often been the pioneers of new techniques and technology. Today such centers are often the main source of teaching at both undergraduate and postgraduate levels. The vast majority of AO faculty work in these centers and many of its members come from them. Because surgeons were selected from lists of AO Alumni members, the previous study (Lifelong Learning) focused largely on the needs of surgeons working in such hospitals. This new study looks at a different population of surgeons: trained consultants working in community hospitals. It investigates whether the needs of these surgeons differ from those working in larger units and explores what the CPD provides do to interact with these surgeons to the benefit of the surgeons and the patients that they serve.

Interviewing surgeons from different cultural backgrounds was initiated to better understand how needs vary in different parts of the world. However, it is impossible to represent the needs of Chinese surgeons and their patients as a whole by interviewing a small number of surgeons from a single city because over 90% of patient care happens outside the hospital system. Similarly, in India the variation in orthopedic practice is huge. Some medical facilities provide the most modern, high-tech treatment for orthopedics problems while, side-by-side, a system of city hospital exists where even the most basic equipment is absent. Clearly the opinion of patients and surgeons will differ if two hospitals are compared.

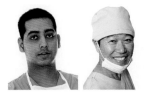

Different cultures

It is impossible to represent the needs of Chinese surgeons and their patients as a whole. Similarly in India the variation in orthopedic practice is huge.

The interpretation of any scientific study is problematic because all studies have their own limitations with regards to validity. In orthopedics and traumatology, quantitative studies have problems with patient selection, outcome measures and follow up. How many articles advocating a particular treatment have proved to be false, as the accumulation of long-term data has shown that the original enthusiasm was based on wrong premises.

Qualitative studies like this one also have their own limitations. We cannot be sure that we asked the "right" questions to the "right" people. Although none of the surgeons who were interviewed had any active connection with the AO Foundation, they all volunteered be interviewed. This group of surgeons does not represent the "average" surgeon, but a group of highly motivated health professionals with an obvious interest in education.

4.1   Why do community hospital surgeons want education?

The main reason why consultant surgeons in community hospitals look for educational help is the same other doctors, regardless of specialty or workplace: trying to solve a clinical problem. All 50 interviewees said that clinical problem solving was *usually* the reason and it was *always* the reason if they needed educational help immediately. These findings are in line with published literature, especially the work of Fox et al [58].

When asked to describe the most recent reason why they looked for educational help, 39 out of 50 respondents described cases with problems relating to trauma. But there was a marked difference between the developed and the developing world: in the developing world all the cases involved acute trauma, in the developed world, 14 of 25 responses related to trauma and 11 to orthopedic problems. These findings support the notion that in the developing world trauma is more important in a mixed orthopedic/trauma practice than it is in the developed world. The data also suggests that educational resources aimed at dealing with acute problems should focus on trauma issues and not those of orthopedic surgery.

The development of new technology was identified as a powerful driver for seeking education, but less so for surgeons working in more specialized units. There was a marked disparity in responses when comparing the developed and developing world. Only 5 of the 25 surgeons from the developing world felt that new technology was an important education driver for them. All were interested in new technology but because they would be unable to introduce it into their hospitals due to financial and logistical constraints they felt that much of those new technologies were irrelevant to their needs. Only twelve of the 25 surgeons from the developed world felt that the introduction of new technology was a major reason why they looked for educational help less than in the previous study. Many of the surgeons stated that they did not feel it was their responsibility to adopt new technologies in their small units.

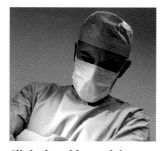

Clinical problem solving
All 50 of the interviewees said that clinical problem solving was usually the reason they looked for educational help and it was always the reason if they needed help acutely.

Just one fifth of the surgeons gave the need to keep themselves generally up-to-date as a reason they looked for education. The numbers that identified this reason were much greater than in the previous Lifelong Learning study (3 out of 147), where most of the surgeons worked in larger units.

4.1.1   Implications for CPD provides

If solving clinical problems is the major reason why surgeons look for educational help then designing educational programs, including events, have to begin with an understanding of these problems. The data from this study strongly supports the concept of "Backward Planning" in curriculum development.

Interview responses suggest that a single course format is not globally applicable when educating consultant surgeons. Since the introduction of new technology differs so widely between the developed and the developing world, the emphasis on new technologies within any given event must be adapted to the target audience. Every needs analysis should examine the ability of surgeons to introduce new technology.

The previous study did not identify the need for a general update in their surgical field as a major educational driver. This study suggests that many consultants working in smaller units need such an update. If this wish is combined with a willingness to get it through a course, then this study supports the idea of courses where participants can select from a list of different topics.

4.2   Does CPD accreditation drive the search for education?

Six of the ten countries involved in the study had detailed, published CPD requirements for surgeons in practice. Two other countries had recommendations published by professional bodies, but adherence to them was not mandatory. Two countries, Israel and Bangladesh had no CPD system at all. CPD requirements affected 41 of the 50 surgeons interviewed yet only two from the UK reported that acquiring CPD points would be a reason for attending an educational event.

There was marked disparity between a country's published CPD regulations and how the surgeons reported it affected them. In three countries that have published CPD requirements half the surgeons either said that no regulations existed or that the regulations did not apply to their situation.

Where a CPD accreditation system existed, most surgeons said that they could easily acquire sufficient points to satisfy the regulatory bodies by attending a small number of meetings. They would never choose to attend an event to pick up points.

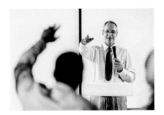

Learning more important
Although many surgeons mentioned the acquisition of CPD points in all countries, collection of CPD points was almost never a reason for attending an educational event or program.

4.2.1   Implications for CPD providers

Systems to ensure that doctors keep their professional skills and know-how up-to-date are installed in many countries. They are almost universal in the developed world and are being introduced in the developing world. Although doctors support the concept of staying up-to-date, this study suggests they do not see current CPD systems as being very important to them. This is reflected in the a marked disparity between the published regulations and the actual behavior of the doctors interviewed.

If CPD accreditation is not that important, then it follows that collecting CPD points is not a critical factor when a surgeon decides to attend an educational event. However, it must be noted that CPD accreditation of educational events constitutes a tight form of quality control and ensures that standards are maintained.

The message from the surgeons is clear. Clinical relevance is much more important than whether an event is accredited for CPD purposes.

4.3   How did surgeons address their most recent clinical problem?

A variety of methods were used by the surgeons to get help in dealing with their most recent clinical problems.

The pattern of initial response was different in the developed and the developing world. Nearly all surgeons in the developed world would use the Internet if they needed information, using a popular search engine like Google. A significant minority of these surgeons used books as their source of information. In the developing world, more surgeons used books to find information. Some surgeons preferred to use books because they felt that they could get information faster than from the Internet. It must be noted that slow or no Internet access was a problem for many and lack of on line information in Chinese was an issue with Chinese surgeons.

When it came to surgical decision making, nearly all the surgeons, whether from the developed or developing world, preferred to discuss cases with colleagues or seniors.

At the same time many of the surgeons encountered problems in their attempt to discuss cases. Many Surgeons working in small units did not have colleagues to discuss cases with, or found it dificult to find someone with the appropriate expertise. Many surgeons also reported that finding time for discussions was difficult because of work pressure. For these reasons many of the surgeons had set up unofficial networks, using the Internet or the telephone. Their contacts were frequently linked to their place of training.

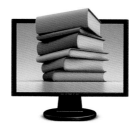

Books and the internet

Nearly all surgeons in the developed countries would use the Internet if they needed information. In the developing world, larger numbers of surgeons used books to gain information.

4.3.1   Implications for CPD providers

The Internet is the preferred source of information for surgeons practicing in the developed world and will probably become so in the developing world as well. The study suggests that many surgeons will not access the special websites unless they appears on the first page of a Google search.

Language is clearly an important issue with regard to distributing information, especially in China.

Although surgeons use books and the Internet to find clinical information, when it comes to problem solving they prefer to discuss cases with someone whose opinion they trust. Surgeons working in community hospitals have more difficulty finding such a person within their own institution than surgeons in larger units. Facilitating professional contacts might be one way in which an educational organization, could improve patient care. This will be discussed further in the section on the Internet.

4.4   How did surgeons working in community hospitals change their practice?

Nearly every surgeon who was interviewed had changed at least one aspect of his practice in the past year (46 out of 50). The driving force behind change was unsatisfactory clinical results. This was often combined with an awareness of new technology. There were no differences between the developed and the developing world.

A variety of information sources were used to incorporate the changes. Commercial websites and workshops organized by pharmaceutical and medical device companies were the single most important educational asset regarding information about new technologies.

Interacting with other surgeons, whether in the hospital or through educational events or conferences, was also an important educational resource.

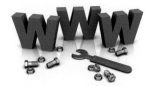

4.4.1   Implications for CPD providers

Although smaller numbers of surgeons in community hospitals say that new technology is an important reason to look for educational assistance, nearly all of them change their clinical practice regularly. If this is related to a new implant, then surgeons in both the developed and developing world find help mostly from implant manufacturers, either company representatives or commercial websites. Even though these websites are clearly labeled as product promotion they represent a huge learning resource to many surgeons worldwide.

Learning through websites
The use of commercial websites and workshops organized by commercial companies was the single most important educational asset with regard to the introduction of new technology.

If surgeons indicate peer discussions are an excellent way to learn about new technology then the providers need to use as much discussion as possible in its courses and it should also consider how this might be continued after an educational event. These findings support the concept of using interactive webinars for teaching new techniques and technologies.

4.5 What were surgeons' best educational experiences?

Overwhelmingly, surgeons said that a personal interaction with a peer or colleague was the best educational experience they ever had. These interactions often occurred during training or fellowship and subsequently many of the surgeons developed an informal network of colleagues with whom they interacted, particularly when they had a difficult case on their hands. These interactions had two striking characteristics: they usually happened as a result of adressing a clinical problem and nearly always invovled a person for whom the surgeon had great regard.

A significant number of surgeons encountered their best ever learning experience while attending an educational event. Practical exercises and talking with experts were given as the main reasons for this. Three surgeons mentioned attending an AO course as their best ever educational experience.

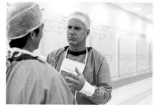

Best educational experience

Overwhelmingly, surgeons said that a personal interaction with a peer or colleague was the best educational experience they ever had. These interactions may have occurred during training or fellowship and subsequently many of the surgeons had developed an informal network of colleagues.

There was no difference in the response patterns between surgeons from developed and developing countries. When compared with the previous Lifelong Learning study data, surgeons from community hospitals had the same response patterns as those working in larger units.

4.5.1 Implications for CPD providers

The opportunity to discuss cases with peers and experts seems to be the most highly valued educational oportunity for surgeons throughout the world regardless of their place of work. If these findings can be extrapolated from the community hospitals studied to the larger surgeon population then personal interaction should be emphasized within all educational events. One can also draw the conclusion that CPD providers should facilitate communication between surgeons either through its existing network or by setting up/ sponsoring communities of practice.

4.6   Did the surgeons use books as references?

Classical textbooks are still very popular with most surgeons. Surgeons stated that they used textbooks to ensure what they are doing is correct. They do it rather to refresh memories than to look for new information. The tendency to use books is more prevalent in developing countries and the data show that older surgeons are slightly more likely to use books than younger ones. It should be noted however, that the oldest surgeon interviewed felt that books were useless and the youngest avoided the Internet if possible.

The books mentioned were all standard orthopedic texts and most surgeons were using old editions, some more than 30 years old. Rockwood and Green's "Fractures in Adults" was by far the most popular trauma textbook (no surgeon interviewed used the AO Principles of Fracture Management, textbook). Many surgeons commented that the extensive reference section in this book was useful.

4.6.1   Implications for CPD providers

Although the Internet is the dominant source of information many surgeons still use books. They tend to use books to confirm their clinical decisions or to refresh their memories rather than to obtain new information.

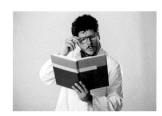

Textbooks still popular

Classical textbooks are still overwhelmingly popular with most surgeons. Surgeons stated that they used books to ensure what they are doing is correct, and to refresh their memories rather than look for new information.

4.7   Were surgeons reading journals?

Journals were read regularly by 11 of the 25 surgeons from developing countries. Three more surgeons commented that they would like to read journals but were unable to do so because of costs. Although most surgeons read selectively, six subscribed to a journal and read it "cover to cover." In the developed world, only six of the interview surgeons interviewed read journals, and they all read articles selectively. It appears there is a marked difference in the use of journals between developed and developing countries. Compared to our previous study, there seems to be greater use of journals by surgeons working in community hospitals than those working in larger units (17 of 50 compared to 19 of 147).

4.7.1   Implications for CPD providers

Reading a journal, even selectively, is far commoner in developing countries than in the developed world. Part of this finding might be explained explained by the fact that in developing countries it is more difficult to access articles through the Internet. Surgeons in the developed world access journal articles by going online, using a search engine and finding relevant articles from a variety of journals. It is clear that research plays a vital part in trauma surgery and that publishing the results is essential to allow this knowledge to be disseminated.

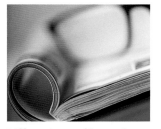

Different use of journals

Reading a journal, even selectively, is far commoner in the developing world than in the developed world. There also seems to be greater use of journals by surgeons working in community hospitals than those working in larger units.

4.8 Did surgeons use the Internet?

All surgeons interviewed used the Internet and, for most of them, it is their preferred source of information. Internet use is more common in the developed countries. Problems with access exist in much of the developing world. There were issues with bandwith, local language and, in China, with censorship of Google and other websites. Missing content in Mandarin also hinders Internet use in China.

Overwhelmingly, the surgeons who wanted information used Google as their preferred search engine. When they were finding out about a specific new technology they logged in to commercial websites where they found good, relevant advice that helped them to apply the new technology.

Of all the Internet media formats the surgeons particularly liked videos, and YouTube was their preferred search engine for this.

Very few surgeons used professional medical websites with the exception of the AO Foundation portal, which was used and valued by 14 of the surgeons interviewed.

4.8.1   Implications for CPD providers
The Internet is the greatest source of information worldwide. Issues exist with access and censorship. Local language can also be a problem. China poses a special challenge because of the large number of surgeons, the rapid expansion of medical services and the limited number of Chinese surgeons who speak English.

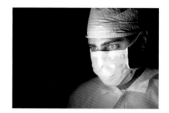

Online videos very popular
Of all the Internet modalities the surgeons particularly liked videos, and remarkably YouTube is their preferred search engine for this. This may be partly due to the fact that videos are multilingual.

4.9 What do surgeons want from the Internet?

All surgeons use the Internet, most of them on a daily basis. Surgeons value the Internet as a source of information.

A significant number of surgeons want to have full access to articles free of charge. There is a demand for more video content on the Internet which relates to surgical techniques, tips and tricks, etc.

Only one surgeon identified "eLearning" as something he would be interested in. One hospital had used compulsory eLearning as a means to ensure that all their medical staff had adequate knowledge of non-accidental injury to children. Because the surgeons interviewed were not confronted with this clinical problem they felt that the eLearning material was very poor. It is likely that this negative reaction was due to a lack of clinical need rather than a poor eLearning module.

Surgeons in community hospitals are especially interested in connecting with experts through the Internet. In the pilot study, three surgeons wished they could ask an expert online if they encountered a problem with a case. Two other surgeons remarked on it when answering the open question "What would you like from the Internet." When asked directly whether they wanted to set up an online community that would allow them to talk to peers and experts, 24 of the 40 respondents were in favor of such a scheme. These surgeons wished to discuss cases on the web, but there were issues with patient confidentiality, who would have access and how to find suitable experts. Trust was thought to be a key factor in peer-to-peer online interactions, but nobody had an idea how this could be achieved.

4.9.1   Implications for CPD providers

Surgeons in community hospitals use and value the Internet as a source of information. Many surgeons would like information available online showing actual surgery, tips and tricks, etc. Such informastion should also include videos.

There are several unanswered questions:

Although most surgeons were keen to use such an online service when proposed, few of them came forward with the idea on their own. How strongly such an idea would be supported is therefore debatable. A pilot online service would be needed to assess the true degree of interest.

All surgeons wanted access to their cases to be limited to a specific group of experts and peers. They did not want to give uncontrolled access to just anybody. But there were differences: some surgeons wanted to give access only to known experts, others wanted to restrict it to surgeons within a geographically defined area, and a third group saw only surgeons with a declared "specialist interest" as users of such an online service. It follows that a "one size fits all" approach to group selection and participation criteria is unlikely to work.

Patient confidentiality is an important issue in the developed world, as is Internet security.

One surgeon raised the question of liability. He asked if he would be held legally liable if he gave online medical advice and the patient suffers as the result of it. Clearly, legal counsel would be needed to assess this risk and any advice may only hold for a single country.

Although the concept of eLearning was known by nearly all the surgeons interviewed, they showed no enthusiasm, despite the potential advantages for surgeons in small hospitals.

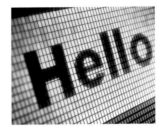

Discussing cases online

One area of interest to surgeons in community hospitals is the ability to interact with experts through the Internet. These surgeons wanted the ability to discuss cases, but there were issues with patient confidentiality and who would get access to the service.

4.10   Do surgeons in community hospitals attend educational events?

Most (43 out of 50) surgeons working in community hospitals like to attend the annual meetings of their societies. These meetings may be organized by national organizations, such as the "Bangladesh Orthopaedic Society", or may be annual yearly conferences of specialized societies, such as "The Hip Society". These annual meetings provide an opportunity to keep up-to-date with the latest research and developments. Our previous study of surgeons working in larger units showed that these were not interested in generalist meetings, but preferred meetings relating to specialist areas of pathology.

These large annual meetings have one main attraction: they cover several topics at the same time and one can choose which speech or seminar to attend. Additionally, surgeons value the possibility to meet and interact with colleagues. These interactions are generally of an informal nature, centered around coffee breaks, lunch and other gatherings. This social aspect of an annual meeting is extremely important, especially in developing countries. (Several surgeons from developing countries took their famiiies to the location of an annual meeting.)

Only two of the surgeons interviewed mentioned attending AO courses. Both of these respondents attended the "Current Concept Master's Course."

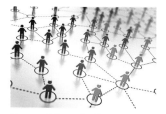

Networking platform

Most surgeons working in community hospitals like to attend the annual meetings of their societies. Surgeons value the ability to interact with their colleagues. The social aspects of annual meetings are extremely important, particularly in the developing world.

4.10.1   Implications for CPD provided

This study shows that the interviewed surgeons in community hospitals rarely attend face-to-face events. Lack of time and money were often cited as reasons, especially in developing countries as other studies initiated by the AO have shown. This study suggests that many of these surgeons see themselves as generalists and like to attend "live" events where there are a number of educational subjects to choose from. Going to large meetings is important to many of these surgeons, particularly in the developing world, because it gives them a chance to meet colleagues to discuss topics they cannot talk about in their own units.

4.11   How important are hospital meetings?

The vast majority of surgeons interviewed attend regular daily hospital meetings. Most of these meetings center around business in connection with acute cases. Community hospitals with staff in training also hold less regular meetings, such as journal clubs, where participants debate recent articles in the scientific literature. These are considered to be useful educational resources. Only three surgeons confirmed that their daily hospital meetings were also attended by other health professionals such as nurses or physiotherapists.

4.11.1 Implications for CPD providers

Meetings are held on a regular daily basis in most hospitals. These meetings mainly relate to the management of acute cases and are usually more business rounds than a teaching session.

The lack of a multi-disciplinary approach to these meetings is remarkable with only three surgeons saying that health professionals other than surgeons were also present. There is certainly room for workplace-based educational projects.

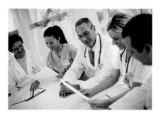

Regular meetings a must

Meetings are held on a regular daily basis in most hospitals. These meetings mainly relate to the management of acute cases and are usually business rounds rather than teaching or learning experiences.

4.12 Do surgeons in community hospitals have problems interacting with their colleagues?

When trying to solve clinical probelms, almost all the interviewed surgeons valued the opportunity to talk with colleagues, peers and seniors. Surgeons in community hospitals work in small groups and the expert advice they seek may not be available within their unit. Many of the surgeons said that their work commitments were so time consuming and strenuous that interaction with colleagues was difficult.

For these reasons, many of the surgeons have created personal informal networks with colleagues which they use when they have a clinical problem.

For example, one surgeon in a developed country had established a network of four local foot and ankle surgeons whom he could refer to for advice. One of the network partners had been his teacher. Relying on past mentorship was a common finding among the surgeons who had set up these informal connections.

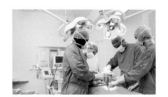

Working in small groups

Surgeons who work in community hospitals work in smaller groups and the expert advice that they seek may not be available within their unit. Many of the surgeons said that their work commitments are so onerous that contact and interaction with their colleagues was difficult.

4.12.1 Implications for CPD providers

This study clearly suggests that surgeons like to discuss clinical problems with other surgeons. In large teaching hospitals where there are many staff and subspecialisation is the rule, surgeons usually can find a suitably qualified expert to talk to. This does not apply to smaller units in community hospitals.

Many surgeons working in smaller units have solved this problem by setting up informal networks with experts and colleagues. The question for any educational organization is whether it could facilitate access to a wider group of fellow surgeons. This is indeed an open-ended question because it could be argued that organically grown networks may be more successful than ones imposed from the outside.

4.13   Are commercial companies of educational help?

Nearly all the surgeons met with commercial representatives on a regular basis. Four surgeons refused to do so unless they themselves initiated contact.Several surgeons mentioned a close relationship with industry representatives. The vast majority of surgeons who had contact with commercial representatives (36 out of 50) thought them to be an extremely useful educational resource, particularly regarding new technology.

Commerical bias was acknowledged but surgeons did not think their decision making was shaped by this. They said it did not influence their choice of implants or techniques, they said.

Sponsorship of educational events by commercial companies seems to be vital in developing countries. Many of these surgeons reported that they rely on commercial sponsorship to be able to attend educational events.

4.13.1   Implications for CPD providers

All independent educational organizations have to ensure that their offerings are scientifically based and free from commercial bias. This study has revealed a paradox: for learning new implant techniques surgeons seem to prefer instruction from commercial sources. Two surgeons explained that they try to look for evidence and discuss things with colleagues before making a change in their surgical practice. However, once they decided to change, they valued the direct approach of commercial sites.

Most surgeons entertain a close relationship with representatives of commercial companies. There were aware of bias, but thought they could handle it without violating principles of patient care.

If surgeons value commercial sites for learning techniques of implant insertion, then providers must consider how to include or link with this information in their own teaching material without compromising ethical values.

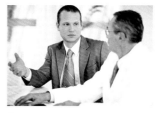

Commerce as resource

Nearly all the surgeons saw commercial representatives on a regular basis. The vast majority of surgeons who did see commercial representatives thought them to be an extremely useful educational resource. They were aware of commercial bias, but did not think that this influenced their decision making.

4.14   Did the surgeons receive any teacher training?

Only four of the surgeons interviewed had received formal training to be teachers. Two of these were ATLS instructors and two had been educated through their Royal Colleges. Those surgeons who had received training felt that this was an important asset both to themselves and the community hospitals in which they worked.

4.14.1   Implications for CPD providers

A very small number of the surgeons interviewed had received training to become better teachers; those who had been trained greatly valued the skills they had acquired. It is impractical for CPD providers to include surgeons from community hospitals in their faculty education programs unless those surgeons become faculty members. Whether online training, in the absence of face-to-face education, would be of use in teaching skills is an open question.

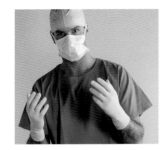

Surgeons as teachers

Only four of the surgeons interviewed had received formal education to be teachers. Those surgeons who had received such training felt that this was an important asset both to themselves and the community hospitals in which they worked.

4.15   Do community hospitals have significant onsite educational resources?

Overwhelmingly, community hospitals do not have significant educational resources. When libraries exist they tend to be small and old fashioned. The major educational resource is an Internet connection, and particularly in the developing countries, this is often slow, making web access difficult.

4.15.1   Implications for CPD providers

The Internet has made the presence of small libraries based in community hospitals obsolete. Surgeons require access to good broadband internet-connection but clearly this is beyond the scope of education providers. The study does support initiatives to make more educational material available through mobile devices such as smart phones and tablet computers.

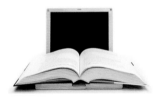

Internet, not libraries

Overwhelmingly, community hospitals do not have any significant educational resources. When libraries exist they tend to be small and old fashioned. The major educational resource is an Internet connection, and particularly in the developing world, it is often slow.

4.16   How community hospitals can improve surgeon education

Surgeons working in community hospitals face special problems. Their need for education is as great, if not greater, than surgeons in larger hospitals, yet they have very little opportunity to interact with professional colleagues.

Teaching hospitals usually set aside time for their consultant staff to teach because teaching is an extremely effective way of learning. The "NationalHealth Service Consultant Contract" specifies that a consultant's work schedule should incorporate some time for teaching. The numbers of staff at teaching hospitals is larger and therefore schedules tend to be less arduous. Time off is easier to arrange so surgeons can attend educational events.

It is not surprising that that interviewees identified one major problem: hospital management often does not recognize how important the education and professional development of surgeons really is. They felt that their employers should invest more resources in surgeon education. In the developed world the issue was lack of time. In developing countries there were problems with financing.

4.16.1   Implications for CPD providers

Surgeons working in community hospitals often cannot afford the time to attend a classic 3–5 day courses. In developing countries these surgeons may not be able to finance such an educational experience. Locally based short update courses, and greater use of webinars and online seminars, show how educational programs can be modified to meet the needs of these surgeons. Such events must be geared towards the demands of the surgeon target audience and the patients served by that group. A course designed for orthopedic surgeons covering a trauma team in Germany is fundamentally different to a course for dedicated trauma surgeons working with limited resources in India, which in turn is different from an event designed for Polish trauma surgeons.

Since interactivity is so valued and many surgeons working in small hospitals feel isolated at times, such events might be followed by an onlineprogram where surgeons can discuss their cases with peers and experts.

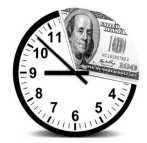

Investing in education

It is not surprising that the main issue identified by the surgeons was that hospital management should recognize the importance of educating their surgeons. In the developed world the investment needed was time. In the developing world there was the additional issue of finances.

4.17   Suggestions for action

There are numerous suggestions, some have already been mentioned above.

In summary they are:

- Always target educational offerings to the clinical needs of surgeons.
- Ensure that the introduction of new technology through education matches clinical needs and availability of equipment/implants in the local community.
- Be aware that many surgeons are primarily orthopedic surgeons who do some trauma and they want a general update on techniques rather than taught cutting edge technology.
- Ensure online information is in the local language.
- Consider using more webinars and videos of clinical cases.
- Work with commercial companies and regulatory bodies to ensure that ethical sponsorship of education can be maintained in developing countries.
- Consider writing a comprehensive trauma textbook to include soft tissue management, conservative treatment, and sports medicine.

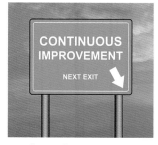

Road map for success

6 References

1 **Davis DA, Thomson MA, Oxman AD, et al** (1992) Evidence for the effectiveness of CME. A review of 50 randomized controlled trials. JAMA; 268(9):1111–1117.

2 **Marinopoulos SS, Dorman T, Ratanawongsa N, et al** (2007) Effectiveness of continuing medical education. Evid Rep Technol Assess (Full Rep); (149):1–69.

3 **Davis D, Galbraith R, et al** (2009) Continuing medical education effect on practice performance: effectiveness of continuing medical education: American College of Chest Physicians Evidence-Based Educational Guidelines. Chest; 135(3 Suppl):42S–48S.

4 **Kumar S, Stenebach M** (2008) Eliminating US hospital medical errors. Int J Health Care Qual Assur; 21(5):444–471.

5 **Wolf FA, Way LW, Steward L** (2010) The efficacy of medical team training: improved team performance and decreased operating room delays: a detailed analysis of 4863 cases. Ann Surg; 252(3):477–85.

6 **Willis CD, Stoelwinder JU, Lecky FE, et al** (2010) Applying composite performance measures to trauma care. J Trauma; 69(2):256–262.

7 **Mahajan RP** (2010) Critical incident reporting and learning. Br J Anesthesia; 105(1):69–75.

8 **de Boer P, Fox R** (2012) Changing Patterns of Lifelong Learning: A study in Surgeon Education. Thieme.

9 **Reeves S, Zwarenstein M, Goldman J, et al** (2008) Interprofessional education: effects on professional practice and health care outcomes. Cochrane Database Syst Rev; (1):CD002213. doi: 10.1002/14651858.CD002213.pub2.

10 **Farmer AP, Legare F, Turcot L, et al** (2008) Printed educational materials: effects on professional practice and health care outcomes. Cochrane database Syst Rev; 16(3):CD004398. doi: 10.1002/14651858.CD004398.pub2.

11 **Davis D, O'Brien MA, Freemantle N, et al** (1999) Impact of formal continuing medical education: do conferences, workshops, rounds, and other traditional continuing education activities change physician behavior or health care outcomes? JAMA; 282(9):867–874.

12 **Davis DA, Thomson MA, Oxman AD** (1995) Changing physician performance. A systematic review of the effect of continuing medical education strategies. JAMA; 274(9):700–705.

13 **Karam MD, Marsh JL** (2010) Does a trauma course improve resident performance on the trauma domain of the OITE? J Bone Joint Surg Am; 92(13):e19. doi: 10.2106/JBJS.J.00368.

14 **Forsetlund L, Bjørndal A, Rashidian A, et al** (2009) Continuing education meetings and workshops: effects on professional practice and health care outcomes. Cochrane Database Syst Rev; (2):CD003030. doi: 10.1002/14651858.CD003030.pub2.

15 **Mehrdad N, Zolfaghari M, Bahrani N, et al** (2011) Learning outcomes in two different teaching approach in nursing education in Iran: e-learning versus lecture. Acta Med Iran; 49(5):296–301.

16 **Young KJ, Kim JJ, Yeung G, et al** (2011) Physician preferences for accredited online continuing medical edu-

cation. J Contin Educ Health Prof; 31(4):241–246. doi: 10.1002/chp.20136.

17 **Fordis M, King JE, Ballantyne CM** (2005) Comparison of the instructional efficacy of Internet-based CME with live interactive CME workshops: a randomized controlled trial. JAMA; 7;294(9):1043–1051.

18 **Casebeer L, Engler S, Bennett N, et al** (2008) A controlled trial of the effectiveness of internet continuing medical education. BMC Med; 6:37. doi: 10.1186/1741–7015-6-37.

19 **Parboosingh IJ, Reed VA, Caldwell Palmer J** (2011) Enhancing practice improvement by facilitating practitioner activity: new roles for providers of continuing medical education. J Contin Educ Health Prof; 31(2):122–127.

20 **American Medical Association. State Medical Licensure Requirements and Statistics,** 2010. http://www.ama-assn.org/resources/doc/med-ed-products/table16.pdf.

21 **General Medical Council** (2012) Continuing professional development: Guidance for all doctors. Accessed July, 23 2013. http://www.gmc-uk.org/CPD_guidance_June_12.pdf_48970799.pdf.

22 **General Medical Council** (2012) Continuing professional development: Guidance for all doctors. Accessed July, 23 2013. http://www.gmc-uk.org/CPD_guidance_June_12.pdf_48970799.pdf.

23 **Glaser B, Strauss A** (1967) The Discovery of Grounded Theory: Strategies for Qualitative Research. Chicago, Aldine Publishing Company.

24 **Glaser B** (1998) Doing Grounded Theory - Issues and Discussions. Mill Valley, Sociology Press.

25 **DentCPD.** Summary of European CPD Regulations by country. http://www.dentcpd.org/workpackages/WP3/WP3-3-Summary-of-European-CPD-regulations-by-country.pdf.

26 **Murgatroyd GB** (2011) Continuing Professional Development: the international perspective. United Kingdom, General Medical Council. http://www.gmc-uk.org/CPD___The_International_Perspective_Jul_11.pdf_44810902.pdf.

27 **de Vries H, Sanderson P, Janta B, et al** (2009) International Comparison of Ten Medical Regulatory Systems:

Egypt, Germany, Greece, India, Italy, Nigeria, Pakistan, Poland, South Africa and Spain. Santa Monica, RAND Corporation. http://www.rand.org/pubs/technical_reports/TR691.

28 **German Medical Association** (2013) Work and training in Germany. http://www.bundesaerztekammer.de/page.asp?his=4.3575.

29 **Schlette S, Klemperer D** (2009) Revalidation of the medical profession in Germany. Euro Observer; 11(2)5–8.

30 **General Medical Council** (2013). Registration and licensing. http://www.gmc-uk.org/doctors/index.asp.

31 **DentCPD.** Summary of European CPD Regulations by country. http://www.dentcpd.org/workpackages/WP3/WP3-3-Summary-of-European-CPD-regulations-by-country.pdf.

32 **Murgatroyd GB** (2011) Continuing Professional Development: the international perspective. United Kingdom, General Medical Council. http://www.gmc-uk.org/CPD___The_International_Perspective_Jul_11.pdf_44810902.pdf.

33 **de Vries H, Sanderson P, Janta B, et al** (2009) International Comparison of Ten Medical Regulatory Systems: Egypt, Germany, Greece, India, Italy, Nigeria, Pakistan, Poland, South Africa and Spain. Santa Monica, RAND Corporation. http://www.rand.org/pubs/technical_reports/TR691.

34 **DentCPD.** Summary of European CPD Regulations by country. http://www.dentcpd.org/workpackages/WP3/WP3-3-Summary-of-European-CPD-regulations-by-country.pdf.

35 **Murgatroyd GB** (2011) Continuing Professional Development: the international perspective. United Kingdom, General Medical Council. http://www.gmc-uk.org/CPD___The_International_Perspective_Jul_11.pdf_44810902.pdf.

36 **The Royal Dutch Medical Association** (2013) http://knmg.artsennet.nl/Over-KNMG/About-KNMG.htm.

37 **Hingstman L, Kenens R, Windt W, et al** (2003) Rapportage Arbeidsmarkt Zorg en Welzijn 2003. [In Report Labor market Care and Welfare]. Volume 48. Tilburg: OSA-publicatie ZW.

38 **Borow M, Levi B, Glekin M** (2013) Regulatory tasks of national medical associations - international comparison

and the Israeli case. J Health Policy Res; 20;2(1):8.

39 **Rowe A, García-Barbero M** (2005) Regulation and licensing of physicians in the WHO European Region. Copenhagen, World Health Organization. Page 73–75. http://www.aemh.org/pdf/RegulandlicencEUphysicians.pdf.

40 **World Health Organization** (2010) Regional Guidelines for Continuing Medical Education (CME)/Continuing Professional Development (CPD) Activities. New Delhi, World Health Organization.

41 **Study in China Admission System (SICAS).** Modern medical education in China. http://www.sicas.cn/Theme/study_Medicine_in_China/Contents_110707144545198.shtml.

42 **Murgatroyd GB** (2011) Continuing Professional Development: the international perspective. United Kingdom, General Medical Council. http://www.gmc-uk.org/CPD___The_International_Perspective_Jul_11.pdf_44810902.pdf.

43 **de Vries H, Sanderson P, Janta B, et al** (2009) International Comparison of Ten Medical Regulatory Systems: Egypt, Germany, Greece, India, Italy, Nigeria, Pakistan, Poland, South Africa and Spain. Santa Monica, RAND Corporation. http://www.rand.org/pubs/technical_reports/TR691.

44 **Chaudhary RR, Naik S, Salhan RN** (2011) Vision 2015. New Delhi, Medical Council of India. http://www.mciindia.org/tools/announcement/MCI_booklet.pdf.

45 **Medical Council of India.** Guidelines for Continuing Medical Education Scheme. http://www.mciindia.org/AboutMCI/CMEProgrammes/GuidelinesforCMEScheme.asp.

46 **Chaudhary RR, Naik S, Salhan RN** (2011) Vision 2015. New Delhi, Medical Council of India. http://www.mciindia.org/tools/announcement/MCI_booklet.pdf.

47 **Medical Council of India.** Guidelines for Continuing Medical Education Scheme. http://www.mciindia.org/AboutMCI/CMEProgrammes/GuidelinesforCMEScheme.asp.

48 **The Times of India** (2011) MCI mulls sending doctors back to school. http://articles.timesofindia.indiatimes.com/2011-04-05/india/29384025_1_mci-cme-credit-conferences.

49 **Gujarat Medical Council.** Continuing Medical Education in Modern Medicine in the State of Gujart. www.gmcgujarat.org/REVISED_CME_GUIDELINES.doc.

50 **World Health Organization** (2010) Regional Guidelines for Continuing Medical Education (CME)/Continuing Professional Development (CPD) Activities. New Delhi, World Health Organization.

51 **Khan AW** (2010) Continuing Professional Development (CPD); What should we do? Bangladesh Journal of Medical Education; 1(1):37–44.

52 **Guinto R** (2012) Medical education in the Philippines: medical students' perspectives. The Lancet;380:S14.

53 **Philippine Medical Association** (2008) Checklist of requirements for accreditation of CPE / CPD providers in accordance with resolution No. 2008-466 series of 2008, Manila, Republic of the Philippines Professional Regulation Commission. https://www.philippinemedicalassociation.org/downloads/circular-forms/CPE-Checklist-of-Requirements-Providers.pdf.

54 **Murgatroyd GB** (2011) Continuing Professional Development: the international perspective. United Kingdom, General Medical Council. http://www.gmc-uk.org/CPD___The_International_Perspective_Jul_11.pdf_44810902.pdf.

55 **Goldstein MS, Donaldson PJ** (1977) Medical education in Thailand: an alternative perspective. Med Educ; 11(3):221–230.

56 **World Health Organization** (2010) Regional Guidelines for Continuing Medical Education (CME)/Continuing Professional Development (CPD) Activities. New Delhi, World Health Organization.